Podiatry Rapid-F
Questions

By Eric Shi, DPM

One of the best ways to retain information is by self-quizzing. When I was a student on externships, one of the hardest things to prepare for were the "pimp questions" I knew I was going to be asked by residents and attendings. In my mind, if I answered every question correctly, I'll look like a stud and earn the program! The honest truth however, is this: *you'll never be able answer every question correctly*. However, this didn't stop me from being as prepared as possible.

I created this list of questions in the middle of externships during my 3rd and 4th year of school. Many of these questions were ones that I got asked on during externships & interviews, others were ones that I created on my own to quiz myself (mostly from material from my other book, <u>Podiatry Student Handbook</u>). I used these questions to quiz co-externs, as well as to quiz myself during any down time when I got tired of reading. What I found most useful was using the voice recorder on my iPhone to record myself reading these questions and then playing them on the car during the many hours I spent driving and stuck in traffic during and between externships—ghetto, I know, but at least it worked!

I know there are many great resources that already exist for podiatry rapid-fire questions, but in my opinion, you can never have too many. **Repetition is key**. I also know that an issue with rapid-fire questions is the credibility of the answer—many of these questions can be answered in different ways based on the source you read. But I did my best to provide the most accurate answers to my knowledge. Regardless, if you find any errors or have any questions, please don't hesitate to email me at <u>pmshandbook@gmail.com</u>.

Happy studying!

Eric Shi, DPM

Podiatry Student Rapid-Fire Questions

Infections and Wound Care

QUESTION	ANSWER
Describe the difference in clinical appearance between a staph vs strep soft tissue infection	**staph**-PURULENCE, localized erythema **strep**-NO purulence, but lymphangitis, soft tissue emphysema
What class of antibiotics is piperacillin?	4th gen PCN
What is tazobactam?	beta lactamase inhibitor
What is the gram stain for clostridium perfringens?	Gram + anaerobe
Describe the dosing for Unasyn and its use	3.0g Q6 IV, broad spectrum or anaerobe
State the dosing for Augmentin and its use	250-500mg PO BID, broad spectrum, anaerobe, enterococcus
What is a terminal syme amputation and its side effects?	AKA distal syme, amputation of lesser digit via racquet-type incision, SE: risk deviation of lesser digits
List some treatments for MSSA soft tissue infection	Penicillin, levaquin, clindamycin
How are PMMA beads made?	combined with bone cement used in OM. the antibiotics used has to be heat labile, broad spectrum, low allergen (gentamycin)
What antibiotic class is clindamycin?	lincosamide
List some side effects of tetracycline	photosensitivity, teeth stain
If a patient has a PCN allergy, name an alternative for Zosyn	Ciprofloxacin
List the drugs found in each generation of cephalosporins, and state which one is anti-pseudomonal	1-cephelexin (keflex), cefazolin (ancef) 2-cefuroxime 3-ceftriaxone, cefotaxime 4-cefepime (pseudomonas) 5-ceftaroline psuedomonas
How is Charcot differentiated from osteomyelitis using ESR/CRP?	Charcot-increase in ESR, not CRP Osteomyelitis-increase in both
What microbe causes erythrasma?	corynebacterium minutissimum
What is the clinical definition of severe sepsis	sepsis + SBP <90 OR SBP drop >40 or lactic acidosis
What is the clinical definition of septic shock	severe sepsis with hypotension despite fluids

Which antibiotics are metabolized by liver?	linezolid, clindamycin, erythromycin, doxycycline
State the dosing for zosyn	3.375g IV Q6 (2.25g renal)
What microbe causes necrotizing fasciitis? How would you treat it?	Strep pyogenes Treat with: vancomycin, zosyn, clindamycin, or 1 million units PEN G
How is osteomyelitis diagnosed on MRI?	T1: hypointense T2: hyperintense
What is the dosing for pre-operative antibiotics? Name 2 for patient with PCN allergy	ancef 2g 1 hr prior to surgery PCN allergy: clinda 900mg Q6 or vanco 15mg/kg
What 3 pathologies appear **green** on wood's lamp?	Microsporum, tinea capitus (bright green), pseudomonas
What are xanthomonas? Proper treatment?	Gram negative bacteria which cause plant diseases, tx with bactrim
Agent responsible for green vs yellow under wood's lamp?	green-pseudomonas yellow-tinea versicolor
Eichenholtz classification XR findings	0-none 1-fragmentation , debris, subluxation 2-resorption, fusion 3-remodeling, decreased sclerosis
Which class of antibiotics is synergistic with aminoglycoside?	Beta lactam
What kind of reaction do you get when you drink alcohol while taking flagyl? Symptoms?	Disulfiram reaction (N/V, tachycardia, SOB)
Inflammatory, proliferative, remodeling phase of wound healing:	1) **Inflammatory**-clotting cascade (platelet, fibrin), vasoconstriction followed by capillary vasodilation 2/2 **HISTAMINE** release, PMN infiltration 2) **Proliferative**-macrophage, collagen, growth factors 3) **Remodeling**-collagen remodeling, **macrophage debride the randomly arranged collagen fibers**
According to the IWGDF classification, what are the diabetic foot risk category chances of re-ulceration	0-N/A 1-2x 2-12x 3-36x
What is the accuracy of the probe-to-bone test based on the Grayson and Armstrong/Lavery articles?	GRAYSON **89% PPV** in severely infected wounds Armstrong/Lavery **57% PPV**, 98% NPV, better test of exclusion

Name the antibiotic that can cause fever	Cephalosporin
Describe the proper technique to take a blood culture	2 sites 20 minutes apart
List the bacteria that most commonly cause skin infections	Staph aureus, GBS
Name the antimicrobial of choice for pseudomonas, and DOC if with PCN allergy	DOC: ciprofloxacin PCN allergy: aztreonam
List 2 antimicrobials of choice for penicillin allergy	Clindamycin or vancomycin
List antimicrobials that treat MRSA	Bactrim, linezolid, daptomycin, doxycycline, clindamycin
Name the antimicrobial that treats vancomycin resitant enterococcus (VRE)	Linezolid (zyvox)
List some examples of Gram + bacteria	Staph strep, enterococcus
Name some antimicrobials to treat enterococcus (2 PO, 2 IV)	Amoxicillin/augmentin (PO), linezolid/vanco (IV)
Name the most common gram negative rod in a diabetic foot infection	Pseudomonas
List as many antimicrobials to treat gram + bacteria	Vanco (IV)/Bactrim (PO) MRSA Cephalosporins-keflex (PO), ancef (IV) Augmentin (enterococcus) Any PCN: Zosyn (pipercillin) Unasyn (ampicillin sulbactam) Clindamycin (PCN allergy) Levofloxacin Azithromycin
List as many antimicrobials to treat gram - bacteria	Fluoroquinolones Aminoglycoside (pseudomonas)
List as many antimicrobials to treat pseudomonas	Ciprofloxacin Aztreonam Fluoroquinolones Aminoglycoside Zosyn cefepime, ceftaroline
What are aminoglycosides used mostly to treat?	Gram negative rod (pseudomonas)
List some examples of aminoglycosides	Gentamycin, tobramycin, amikacin
What are fluoroquinolones used mostly to treat?	Gram negatives (pseudomonas)
What is aztreonam used mostly to treat?	Pseudomonas (**for PCN allergy**)

What causes red NECK syndrome?	rifampin
Describe the mechanism of action of a macrolide vs aminoglycoside	Macrolide-binds to 50s ribosomal unit Aminoglycoside-binds to 30s ribosomal unit
List 2 antimicrobial treatments for C diff	Vanco PO or flagyl PO
What type of diarrhea is due to long-term use of antibiotics?	C diff pseudomembranous colitis
List 3 antimicrobial treatments for anaerobe What if PCN allergy?	Augmentin PO, unasyn/zosyn IV PCN allergy: Flagyl, clinda, cipro,
What bacteria is associated with salt water?	Vibrio vulnificus
Name the microbe and drug of choice for gas gangrene	**Microbe**: group A strep (GAS) or clostridium perfringens **Drug of choice**: PEN G, clindamycin
List some side effects of aminoglycosides	Nephrotoxicity/ototoxicity —> non reversible
Name the drug of choice for a salt water wound injury	Doxycycline
Name a gram negative anaerobe rod	Bacteriodes fragilis
Describe how to interpret sensitivity chart to know if the staph is MRSA and if hospital/non hospital acquired	MRSA = oxacillin resistant hospital acquired = Bactrim resistant
Describe what the pus of clostridium perfringens look like	dishwater bubble
Name the most common microbe for grafts or hardware	staph epidermitis
Name 2 agents used in WBC tag scans	indium and gallium
What is type 3 diabetes known as?	gestational during pregnancy
What level glucose would lead to poor wound healing?	>250
What is DM1?	AKA IDDM Body does not produce insulin Destroyed pancreatic islet cell
What is DM2?	NIDDM Cells insulin resistant, hyperinsulinemia
What is diabetes insipidus?	SIADH Lack of ADH, kidneys unable to conserve water
Describe the Frykberg classification	1-FF 2-TMT 3-midfoot 4-ankle 5-calcaneus

Neurology System

QUESTION	ANSWER
Stages of Charcot (Eichenholtz classification)	0-inflammatory 1-developmental 2-coalescent 3-remodeling
Theories of Charcot	1) neurotraumatic (German) 2) neurovascular (French) 3) combination
What to cut when doing dorsal approach neuroma	Deep Transveerse Metatarsal Ligament (DTML)
3 types of CMT	CMT1: demyelinating CMT2: axon degeneration CMT3: Dejerine Sottas Dz
MC causes of Charcot	DM, syringomyelia, tabes dorsalis
How to definitively dx CMT	1) EMG/NCV 2) Nerve biopsy: **onion bulb formation**—axons with layers of demyelinating and remyelinating Schwann cells, axonal degeneration
Charcot Marie Tooth (CMT) disease causes what foot shape	Cavus
Cerebral palsy causes what foot deformity?	Equinus
Causes of diabetes?	"DANGTHERAPIST" diabetes, alcohol, nutrition B12, guillan barre, trauma, hereditary CMT, endocrine (thyroid), radiculopathy, polio, infection HIV, sarcoidosis
What is Baxter's nerve	First branch of lateral plantar along N medial ankle, hugs medial tubercle
Describe the neuropathic pattern of DM neuropathy	"stocking glove" distribution
3 parts of Babinski sign	hallux DF, fanning of toes, flexion of leg and thigh
What is Sullivan's sign	splay toe due to neuroma
What is Gauthier's test	squeeze MT head and ROM the MT
What is Phalen's maneuver for foot	invert and PF
What are the 3 most common causes of CMT disease?	DM, syringomyelia (spinal cord cyst), tabes dorsalis

Describe the difference between CRPS 1 vs CRPS 2	CRPS1-absence of nerve damage, AKA **RSD** CRPS2-WITH nerve damage 2/2 trauma, AKA **causalgia**
At what age does Charcot-Marie-Tooth disease present?	30 yo-autosomal dominant 8 yo-autosomal recessive
Describe the MRI results for Charcot vs osteomyelitis	marrow edema across multiple bones (Charcot) **single bone (osteo)**
Describe the Sunderland classification for nerve injury	1) neuropraxia 2) axonotmesis 3) disruption of fascicle organization 4) partial severance 5) neurontmesis
What is the mechanism of a Bier block?	IV anesthetic injection would block adjacent nerve
Describe the dermatome innervation for the posterior leg	lateral S1, medial S2
Describe the dermatome innervation for the anterior foot	Medial hallux L4 (knee), middle digits L5, lateral S1
What is the pathophysiology of multiple sclerosis?	patchy demyelination, **optic neuritis** (BLINDNESS),
What are the physical symptoms of multiple sclerosis?	EXACERBATED BY HEAT, bladder dysfunction, Charcot triad: 1) nyastagmus 2) scanning speech (syllables separated by pauses) 3) intention tremor
What is another name for ALS? What are its physical exam findings?	Lou Gehrig disease, an upper/lower motor neuron disease HYPER-REFLEXIA deep-tendon reflexes on physical exam
What are some symptoms associated with Guillain Barre?	AKA Landry's paralysis, precipitated by infection Drop foot, risk death via respiratory paralysis
What age would Charcot Marie Tooth present in an autosomal recessive vs autosomal dominant genetic pattern?	recessive-age **8** dominant-age 30, MORE COMMON
Friedreich's ataxia affects which age group? What is its main cause of death?	scoliosis in childhood Death by CARDIAC complications
Describe the stages of type 1 CRPS AKA reflex sympathetic dystrophy (RSD)	**Red**-acute days-weeks **White**-dystrophic cyanotic 3-6 months **Blue** atrophic waxy >6 months

EMG	**normal**-at rest, silent **denervation**-fasciculations at rest, **DEC # motor units** INC amplitude and duration due to collateral sprouting of new nerves
What is the normal value for nerve conduction velocity studies?	>40mps
What is the mechanism in using alcohol for nerve sclerosis in the treatment of neuromas?	dehydrates, shrinking Wallerian degeneration

Vascular System

QUESTION	ANSWER
Monckeberg's sclerosis is found in in what layer of the blood vessel?	tunica media
What are some types of endovascular stents?	drug eluting, bare metal
What are some differential diagnoses for leg pain?	DVT, rhabdomyolysis, compartment syndrome, nec fasc
What is Turk's test	AKA Perthe's tourniquet test, compress superficial vv if blood moves from deep to superficial, deep valve is incompetent
"Triad" of clinical symptoms found in pulmonary embolism?	hemopytsis, SOB, chest pain
What is the difference between erythema vs purpura?	**erythema**-dilated capillary, blanchable **purpura**-hemorrhagic lesion, non blanchable
Presentation of foot pain in arterial vs venous disease	arterial-pain relieved with dependancy venous-pain relieved with elevation
What casues Raynaud's phenomenon?	paroxsymal vasospasm due to cold or stress
How many millimeters of mercury is good for compression stocking?	35-40mmHg
What is Buerger's disease	small/medium angiopathy, due to hypersensitivity to tobacco
Manage heparin s/p DVT by keeping PTT at which value?	PTT 2x normal (40-60)
List the stages of arterial occlusion	1) intermittent claudication <0.8 2) rest pain (night) <0.5 3) gangrene

What TcPO2 associated with healing wounds	>55mmHg
List some examples of stasis in Virchow's triad	CHF, MI, obesity, arrhythmias
List some examples of hypercoagulability in Virchow's triad	factor V leiden, neoplasm, pregnancy, surgery, polycythemia vera
What range of TCPO2 is healing uncertain?	30-55mmHg
Describe arteriosclerosis obliterans	proliferation of **intima**, symptoms similar to PAD
Describe thromboangitis obliteratans	AKA Buergers disease hypersensitivity to smoking
Arterial embolism MC source, and site	**Source**: heart **Site**: femoral A
What causes thrombosis and what is its treatment?	Forming a clot, hx of atherosclerosis, tx with TPA
What is the gold standard method to diagnose DVT?	venography
Describe the difference between erysipelas and cellulitis	**Cellulitis** involves dermis and subcutaneous fat, **Erysipelas** is more superficial than cellulitis, dermis and superficial lymphatics
What does TcPO2 measure?	microangiopathy

Dermatology System

QUESTION	ANSWER
Frostbite stages	1) no blister 2) clear blister 3) hemorrhagic blister 4) full thickness
What are the distinct features of pyoderma gangrenosum? What is the treatment?	purple overhanging edge, associated with inflammatory conditions such as IBS, ulcerative colitis, Crohn's. Treat with topical steroids
What skin CA to rule out in venous stasis wound	Squamous cell carcinoma
What is ecythma	impetigo extending to DERMIS under crusted surface infection
What fungus causes vesicular tinea pedis	T. mentagrophytes
What is chilblains?	Erythematous, recurrent skin lesion 2/2 cold with similar appearance to cellulitis
What causes trench foot?	Prolonged immersion in cold/cool water

Degrees of burns, timing?	**First**-epidermis (5-10 days) **Second**-does NOT penetrate dermis (10-60 days) **Third**-thru dermis (no healing, no sensation)
List the 4 types of melanoma Which is located in palms and soles? Which has the worst prognosis? Which is described as melanotic whitlow? Which involves Hutchinson's sign?	**superficial spreading** (MC), wide before deep **nodular** (WORST prognosis), ulcerate, colorful **lentigo** (slow, elderly, least metastasize) **acral** (melanotic whitlow-palms, soles, Hutchinson, Blacks, palms and soles)
Melanoma staging? (Clark's levels)	1-superifical 2-basement 3-papillary 4-reticular 5-subcutaneous
Causes of skin graft failure?	hematoma, lack of vascularization, infection, inadequate immobilization
Skin conditions often associated in diabetics vs patients with venous insufficiency	**DM**-necrobiosis lipoidica diabeticorum **venous stasis**-LDS lipodermatosclerosis (inverted champagne)
What is the skin lesion associated with Reiters disease?	keratoderma blennorrhagicum
What orientation are resting skin tension lines (RSTL) on the plantar foot	transverse
How long does it take for basal cells to reach the skin surface?	1 month
What are the 2 layers of dermis and the structures found in each?	**papillary** 1/3 meissener's corpuscles (touch) **reticular** 2/3 pacinian corpuscles (vibratory)
Describe the eccrine gland: secretion, location, and control	Secretion: watery secretion Location: palms/soles Control: sympathetic
Describe the apocrine gland: secretion, location, and control	Secretion: viscous, sticky odorous, Location: areola, pubis and perineum Control: adrenergic
Describe the sebaceous gland: secretion, location, and control	Secretion: sebum/oil Location: lubricates hair follicle, holocrine gland, Control: puberty controlled by androgens
Define a macule	Flat lesion <1cm
Define a patch	Flat lesion >1cm
Define a papule	Raised lesion <1cm
Define a plaque	raised lesion <1cm
Define a nodule	firm lesion <1cm

Define a tumor	firm lesion >1cm
Define a vesicle	Fluid filled lesion <0.5cm
Define a bullae	fluid filled lesion >0.5cm
Define a cyst	Non-infected deep fluid
Define a burrow	tunnel 2/2 to parasite
Define a wheal	AKA hives, elevated then disappears
Define a pustule	vesicle or bulla filled with pus
Define scales	flaking epidermis
Define lichenification	thickening leathery 2/2 scratch
Define an excoriation	deep excoriation not breaching dermis
Define a crust	dried debris
Define a scar	cicatrix fibrous connective tissue replacing dermis
What is diascopy?	glass slide test erythema-blanch, purpura-hemorrhagic lesions
In a KOH test, what is the purpose of KOH?	KOH disolves keratin
What is the Nikolsky sign?	rubbing results in exfoliation seen in bulls pemphigus, diabeticorum
A shave biopsy samples what skin layer?	epidermis only
A punch biopsy samples what skin layer?	**full thickness** no need to suture up 2mm
At what size is an excisional biopsy indicated?	>8mm, used for dermal and SC cyst, malignant melanoma
What is a Tzanck test used for?	viral disease (herpes). Fix with Wright's stain multinucleate giant cell = pos test
How does tinea capitis appear on wood's lamp? How does pseudomonas appear on wood's lamp?	Bright/light green Regular green-psuedomonas
How does tinea versicolor appear on wood's lamp?	yellow gold
What does hypopigmentation on wood's lamp indicate?	ash leaf macule (tuberous sclerosis)
Contact dermatitis, AKA (2)? Mediated by what? Location? Examples?	AKA ECZEMA or DELAYED cutaneous hypersensitivity T-cell mediated, FLEXOR surface

Irritation vs allergic	**1) irritation**-first time (detergents, fiberglass) **2) allergic**-exposure sensitizes to future (POISON IVY, RUBBER, NICKEL)
What is atopic dermatitis? Describe 3 types	Hereditary, predisp lowered threshold to itching flexoral surface **infantile**-face **childhood**-antecubital/popliteal fossa **adult**-shrink
Treatment for atopic dermatitis	inc AERATiON
What is urticarial?	AKA hives, pruritic wheals that disappear
What causes nummular discoid eczema?	coin shaped plaque, bacterial infection
Describe dishidrotic eczematous dermatitis (dyshidrosis)	Reaction to **METALS, not sweat** vesicles appear like tapioca on SOLES
Describe seborrheic dermatitis	AKA **cradle cap**, HIV, greasy yellow scale rash FOREHEAD
Describe the appearance of impetigo and its cause	staph aureus, yellow honey crust
Describe the appearance of pitted keratolysis. What is its cause?	pitting of stratum corneum (on the sole of the foot) moth-eaten due to bacterial keratolytic enzyme
Which fungus causes tinea capitus?	Tinea tonsurans
How is a wart clinically differentiated from callus?	wart-pain with lateral pressure, spongy PUNCTATE bleeding center, absence of skin lines callus-skin lines present, pain with direct pressure
Mollucusm contagiosum is caused by which virus?	pox virus
Herpetic whitlow is located where?	distal phalanx
Ramsay hunt's syndrome affects which nerve?	face and auditory nerve
What pathology is the "dimple sign" associated with?	Dermatofibroma Treatment: excision with pathological exam They are common benign tumors but can be confused with pigmented BCC and melanomas can
Cavernous hemangioma is associated with which syndrome? What is its XR finding? Color of skin discoloration?	Maffuci's syndrome, XR calcification, BLUE discoloration PAIN, RAPID INCREASE IN SIZE Tx: surgical excision
What is the thickness of the epidermis?	0.04mm

What is the thickness of the dermis?	0.5mm
What layer does scabies lay eggs in	corneum
Syphilis stages	1-painless 2-painful 3-neurosyphyllis (gumma)

Nail Pathology

QUESTION	ANSWER
For nail matrixectomy procedures, what are concentrations of NaOH, acetic acid, phenol	NaOH-10%, acetic acid-5%, phenol-89%
What is Hutchinson's sign of the nail?	1) pigmentation of proximal nail fold indicative of subungual melanoma OR Bowen's disease (benign)
Subungual hematoma level treatments	>25% remove nail, <25% trephinate
What is Beau's line?	transverse horizontal depression associated with nail trauma, growth arrest MI, PE, fever
What is Mee's line?	Transverse white discoloration 2/2 arsenic poisoning
What is the XXXngula labia known as?	Medial or lateral nail fold
What causes blue nail?	Antimalarials (minocycline), Wilson's disease
What causes brown nail?	Addison's disease
What is koilonychia?	spoon nail due to iron deficiency anemia,
What is Lindsay nail?	half pink and white. Liver disease
What is Muehrcke's nail?	transverse white band, nephrotic syndrome
Onychopuntata	pitting
Onychorrhexia	brittle nail
Onychotillomania	picking at nail
Red lunula may be a sign of what medical condition?	CHF
Splinter hemorrhage may be a sign of what medical condition?	bacterial endocarditis
Describe the appearance of Terry's nail	proximal white distal red

List some surgical nail procedures	**Frost**-inverted L
	Winograd-suture skin to nail
	Suppan-surgically resect matrix

Bone Disease & Tumors

QUESTION	ANSWER
What are 2 types of primary repair in bone healing?	1. Cutting cone (parallel to fx line)
	2. gap healing (perpendicular)
For an 8 yo who presents with a pathological tibial fracture, you are worried about what tumor?	Osteosarcoma
Which bone tumor would you see the "fallen fragment sign"	UBC
Name the most common benign bone tumor in children	non ossifying fibroma
How can smoking delay bone healing?	nicotine and vasoconstriction
	carbon monoxide and binding to O2
At what age does when does Sever's fuse	15 yo
Which phase of bone healing is the longest?	Remodeling (70% of entire process)
What is gap healing?	Primary healing, bone deposition 90 degrees to orientation of bone frag
Most common soft tissue mass in the foot?	Ganglion cyst
Osgood Schlatter is OCD of what bone?	tibial tuberosity
Blount's disease is OCD of what bone?	proximal tibial epiphysis
What is the crescent sign in AVN? This is found in which stage of the Smilie classification?	lateral projections, Smilie stage 3
Smillie classification	1) epiphysis fracture 2) central depression 3) lateral projections 4) projection fx 5) flattened
MC soft tissue in body?	lipoma
zones in growth plate	zone of growth
	zone of maturation
	zone of transformation
What is Ilfeld's disease?	agenesis of fibular sesamoid

What disease increases fat pad thickness?	acromegaly
Bone lesions found in the calcaneus	Intraosseus **lipoma**, ABC, UBC, GCT, ewing's, chondrosarcoma, chondroblastoma
A 12 yo who presents with thigh pain most likely has which bone disease?	Slipped capital femoral epiphysis
Kohler's **age**, location	3-6, osteochondrosis of navicular
What is Iselin's disease?	Osteochondrosis of base 5th MT
What is the Smillie classification?	1) epiphysis fracture 2) central depression 3) lateral projections 4) projection fx 5) flattened
2 types of non-union	**Hypertrophic**-elephant/horse foot **Atrophic**
Which organs do synovial sarcoma metastasize to?	Lungs, bones, lymph nodes
Lytic bone tumors	FOGMACHINES Fibrous dysplasia, osteoblastoma, giant cell, myeloma, ABC, chondroblastoma, hyperPTH, infection, nonossifying fibroma, enchondroma, solitary/UBC
Describe primary vs secondary bone healing	**Primary**-rigid fixation, cutting cone mechanism (osteoclast and osteoblast activity) **Secondary**-hematoma, soft callus, hard callus
What is the "coin sign"/ "coin on edge" / "silver dollar sign"	Kohler's disease-osteochondrosis of navicular
What is the crescent sign indicative of?	AVN
What is heterotopic ossification?	formation of bone in tissues which normally don't have it.
What are the effects of smoking on bone healing?	1) nicotine leading to vasoconstriction 2) carbon monoxide binds to O2
What part from the proximal tibia would an autograft be taken?	Gerdy's tubercle
What are Glissane's bony fusion principles	1) remove cartilage 2) appositon 3) position 4) maintain apposition
What is the rule of 1/3's for cortical thickness	normal for age <40 1/3 for near and far cortex, 1/3 for medullary canal rule of 1/4 for age >40

What is the piezogeneic effect?	similar to dynamization, stress generates electric potentials in bone resulting in callus formation
What are the zones of the epiphyseal growth plate? What are their functions?	**Proliferation**-chondrocyte production **maturation**-chondrocyte growth **transformation**-calcification of chondrocyte **provisional** calcification-border of metaphysis
What are the phases of bone healing?	inflammatory, hematoma, reparative/regenerative (soft and hard callus), remodeling
What is rarefaction?	Decreased density of bone similar to periosteal reaction
What are the patterns of destruction found in bone?	geographic—>moth eaten—>permeative
What are the types of periosteal reaction?	buttressing—>lamellate (onion skin)—>sunburst—>hair on end (spiculated)
Most common malignant tumor	multiple myeloma
Diaz/Mouchet osteochondrosis of which bone?	Osteochondrosis of Talus
Thiemann's osteochondrosis of which bone?	Osteochondrosis of phalanges
Lewin osteochondrosis of which bone?	Osteochondrosis of distal tibia
Ritter osteochondrosis of which bone?	Osteochondrosis of proximal fibular head
Treve osteochondrosis of which bone?	Osteochondrosis of fibular sesamoid
Renandier osteochondrosis of which bone?	Osteochondrosis of tibial sesamoid
Lance osteochondrosis of which bone?	Osteochondrosis of cuboid
Assmann osteochondrosis of which bone?	Osteochondrosis of 1st MT head
Buschke osteochondrosis of which bone?	Osteochondrosis of cuneiform
Mueller Weiss osteochondrosis of which bone?	Adult osteonecrosis of navicular
What is the typical clinical presentation of a patient with Freiberg's infraction?	young female athlete with MT pain
Most common osteochondrosis, location?	Legg Calve Perthes disease, femoral head
What are the stages of Paget's disease?	1. osteoclast 2. mixed 3. osteoblast 4. malignant degeneration
Difference between lamellar vs woven bone?	woven-unorganized, weak lamellar-organized, strong

Contact vs gap healing	BOTH are types of primary bone healing **contact**-cutting cone tip haversion remodeling, lamellar bone **gap healing**-hematoma, woven bone
What is Brodie's abscess?	lytic lesion surrounded by sclerotic rim
At what age does Sever's apophysitis present?	8-12 yo, resolves when apophysis fuses to calcaneal body
Phases of bone graft healing	1. vascular ingrowth 2. osteogenesis 3. osteoinduction 4. osteoconduction 5. remodeling
Where is a unicameral bone cyst (UBC) found?	calcaneus
Most common benign bone tumor in children	non ossifying fibroma
What do you see in in a foot XR for a patient with pseudohypoparathyroidism?	BRACHYMETATARSIA Brachymetatarsia could also be due to Down syndrome, Turner's,
Paget's disease also known as? Laboratory findings?	osteitis deformans lab: inc alk phos but normal Ca2+/phosphate
What is Gardner's syndrome?	Multiple **osteomas**, polyposis of large bowels
Osteoma location? XR findings?	**Skull, periosteum** XR finding: osteochondroma w/o cartilaginous cap
Location of ossifying fibroma? Location of non ossifying fibroma/fibrocortical defect?	**Ossifying fibroma**: related to fibrous dysplasia (ground glass) **MANDIBLE** **Non ossifying/fibrocortical defect**: muscle/tendon insertion, connective tissue, **Fibrocortical defect**: <4cm
Chondroblastoma appearance? Location?	mimic ABC (hemorrhagic changes) **epiphysis**
Tumor found at the epiphysis?	Chondroblastoma
Tumor found intracortical?	Non ossifying fibroma & ossifying fibroma
Tumor found at the periosteum?	Osteoma
What is Shepherd's crook?	**Fibrous dysplasia** leading to varus bowing of femur
What is Codman's triangle?	triangular elevation of periosteum, seen in osteosarcoma

MC primary benign tumor	osteochondroma
MC malignant primary tumor	multiple myeloma, osteosarcoma
Name 2 common malignancies in pediatrics	Ewing's, osteosarcoma
List the MC sources of cancer that can end up at foot	prostate, breast, kidney, thyroid, lung
List some malignant bone tumors	osteosarc, chondrosarc, fibrosarc, ewing's sarc, multiple myeloma
What is an enostosis?	bone island
Describe characteristics of an osteoblastoma	AKA giant osteoid osteoma, AKA osteogenic fibroma **pain NOT relieved by aspirin**
Osteosarcoma occurs during which age group?	teenager during growth spurt
Describe the characteristics of an enchondroma	(proximal) phalanges resembling bone cyst
What is Ollier's disease?	MULTIPLE enchondroma (enchondromatosis)
What is Maffucis syndrome?	enchondromas associated with **soft tissue hemangioma and telangiectasia, poor prognosis**
Describe the appearance of chondroblastoma. Location?	mimic ABC (hemorrhagic changes) located at **epiphysis**
Describe the characteristics of a giant cell tumor	**fibrohistocytic**: connective tissue, stromal, giant cell, SOAP BUBBLE appearance
Describe the characteristics of a UBC	**fallen fragment sign**-bone frag falls into cyst, calcaneus
Describe the characteristics of an aneurysmal bone cyst (ABC)	Fluid fluid levels, blood filled cyst
Describe the characteristics of Ewing's sarcoma	Children <20 yo, M>F Caucasians, MOST LETHAL primary bone lesion Small blue-cell tumor
Describe the characteristics of a brown tumor	hyperPTH, osteoclastoma. Holes in bone filled with osteoclast fibrous tissue
Describe the characteristics of an osteoid osteoma	"NIDUS", Oval radioluceny surrounded by sclerosis TIBIA AND FEMUR
What tumor is located at the epiphysis?	Chondroblastoma
What tumor is located intracortically?	Non ossifying fibroma & ossifying fibroma
What tumor is located at the periosteum?	osteoma

What is the maximum distance between fracture site to still allow for bone healing?	1cm or **>1/2 diameter bone**
What is a pseudoarthrosis?	end stage of nonunion, fibrocartilaginous surface with synovial fluid
describe 4 different atrophic nonunions	**Torsion wedge**-intermed fragment healed to one of the main frag but not the other **Comminuted**-necrotic intermed fragment **Defect**-loss of fragment, large gap **Atrophic**-end result
Describe the mechanism for bone stimulators	Electronegative charge stimulates bone growth
Describe cortical bone healing	weakest at 8 wks, Haversian system RADIOLUCENT when healing
Describe cancellous bone healing	RADIODENSE when healing, REPLACED by new bone STRONGER each week
What is "creeping substitution"?	graft cells replaced by viable bone
What is osteoinduction?	BMP to induced mesenychmal cells —> osteoblast
What is Haversian remodeling?	Primary bone healing via cutting cone, simultaneous remodeling and formation of bone In CORTICAL bone
What are some radiographic findings in rickets?	bowing, looser zone, milkman zone, metaphyseal cupping, fraying. 2/2 vit D def **osteoid seam**-lines of unmineralized bone appear as pseudofx
What are some radiographic findings in scurvy?	transverse line of inc density "white line of Frankel" with adjacent dark **scurvy line**, trummerfield zone
What is the radiographic finding of a ring epiphysis in scurvy called?	Wimburger's sign
What is the radiographic finding of a beaky outgrowth scurvy called?	Pelken's spur
What are some XR findings for acromegaly?	soft tissue thickening (fat pad), large heel spur, narrow proximal phalanx shaft
How do osteochondromatosis form?	when piece of growth plate breaks off during childhood, disease of cartilage, can —> chondrosarcoma
What are some XR findings of osteogenesis imperfecta?	severe osteopenia (trabeculae in MT head),

	gracile (**narrow girth**) tubular bones
Describe the radiologic findings of Paget's disease	BOWING, excess resorption/remodeling, near joint towards diaphysis
What is the radiological pathognomic sign found in Paget's disease?	"blade of grass" or "flame" sign (active mixed osteoclast/blast stage)
What is a radiographic finding for fibrous dysplasia?	ground glass
What is another name for osteopetrosis? Describe the XR findings	aka marble bone disease, bone within bone appearance
Describe melorheostosis	wax flowing down candle (wavy inside OR outside cortex)
At what age do sesamoids ossify?	8 yr
At what age do the posterior calcaneus, post talus, base 5th fuse?	post calc-15 yo base 5th-15 yo post talus-18 yo
In what disease does the radiographic bone age does NOT match actual age?	hypothyroidism (cretinism)
What is myositis ossificans?	ossification of muscle, can be post traumatic
What is a phlebolith?	rice shape calcification 2/2 chronic venous dz
Describe the radiographic difference between rarefaction vs eburnation	**Rarefaction**: decreased density **Eburnation**: Subchondral sclerosis 2/2 erosion
What is the 4th phase of bone scan used for?	Patients with poor blood flow, PVD, DM takes 24 hrs
What is the 15% rule in regards to XR optical density	increasing kVp by 15% OR double mA would make image more dark (optical density) 30% change in optical density necessary to notice change
What is the effect of increasing source-to-image-distance (SID) on image sharpness?	Increases
What is the effect of increasing object-to-image-distance (OID) on image sharpness?	Decreases
Radiographic distortion is caused by what?	UNEQUAL magnification, i.e. a circle shot at an angle would appear as an oval
What is the purpose of the grid in an XR machine?	picks up scatter XR to make XR more sharp, must inc mA to compensate
What is the purpose of FIXING?	removes UNBOUND silver using hypo (thiosulfate)

What is the definition of the angle of gait and and base of gait?	Angle of gait-feet angled at 15 degrees Base of gait-feet 2 inches apart
Does MRI produce radiation?	no ionizing radiation
What is X-ray fog?	Artifact where unintentional exposure 2/2 reducing contrast, scatter radiation, LIGHT LEAK MC
What are some early vs late gout XR findings?	Early: NONE (joint sparing) l Late: jt destructive

First Ray, Forefoot Pathology & Arthridities

QUESTION	ANSWER
1mm wedge in a closing bas wedge ostoetomy (CBWO) corrects how many degrees of IMA?	3 degrees
What are the steps in performing a McBride procedure?	Medial capsulotomy, exostectomy, cut DTMTL, release adductor, fibular sesamoidectomy
Name the best type of screw to fixate the osteotomy in for bunion correction	cancellous screw-COMPRESSION
What is the purpose of 1st MPJ implant?	relieve pain, NOT to restore normal ROM
Describe the structures cut in a lateral release	adductor tendon, transverse MT ligament, lateral capsulotomy, fibular sesamoid ligament
Describe the biomechanical mechanism of action for the chevron osteotomy	restoration of IMA leads to windlass leads to stable first ray
List some joint destructive procedures for the 1st MTPJ	keller, stone (coronal slice), mayo (rounded slice), arthroplasty, arthrodesis
List the etiologies for hallux limitus	hypermobile 1st ray aka overpronation MPE long/short 1st MT posttraumatic arthropathy
Which base wedge procedure does not shorten 1st MT?	crescentic (OBWO)
What is the 1st MTPJ ROM to diagnose hallux limitus?	<65 degrees
List some shaft procedures for HAV. Describe the is Kalish procedure	scarf, ludloff, mao, lambrinudi kalish (chevron with long dorsal arm)

List some base procedures for HAV	lapidus, crescentic, juvara, loison balacescu, logroscino
List some joint destructive procedures for hallux limitus	keller, stone (head resection), mayo (crescentic head resection) fusion (mckeever)
List some joint preserving procedures for hallux limitus	kessel bonney, watermann, waterman green, youngswick, regnauld (mexican hat)
Describe the Root Orien and Weed stages of HAV	1-subclinical subluxation of 1st MTPJ (lat shift of prox phalanx) 2-hallux abducts 3-met primus varus deformity 4-subluxation/dislocation of 1st MTPJ
List some neck procedures for hallux valgus	Hohmann, Mitchell, Peabody, Wilson, DRATO
How does staking the head lead to hallux varus?	FHB and abductor hallucis allowed to dominate especially in the absence of adductor hallucis
What is a Morton's foot?	Short first MT
What vein to watch out for in when performing Lapidus procedure?	medial marginal vein medially or deep perforating artery in Intermetatarsal space
Describe these following procedures: Waterman, Waterman Green, Youngswick, Kessel and Bonney	All surgical procedures for hallux limitus, all with cheilectomy Waterman-DFWO of MT neck Waterman Green-waterman preserving sesamoids Youngswick-Austin with dorsal wedge removed Kessel and Bonney-DFWO base of proximal phalanx
How much does 1mm shift of capital fragment correct?	1 deg IMA
Common cause for hallux varus	Removal fibular sesamoid, staking head, congenitally flat MT head, trauma, overcorrection of IMA
List some complications from the Keller procedure	floppy toe cock up toe metatarsalgia 2/2 to losing hallux purchase
Mayo block	1st MT base, 1st IM space blocks: medial dorsal cut, saphenous, deep peroneal, common plantar digital, proper plantar digital
Reiter's syndrome symptoms?	"Can't see can't pee can't climb a tree" (arthritis, urethritis, uveitis)

What type of graft used in lapidus	Shear strain relieved graft-pack graft dorsally at 1st MT cuneiform joint
What screws are used for Lapidus? Where do the screws cross?	**3.5 or 4.0 screw** HR screw 1st MT base to med cuneiform Cross in base of 1st MT
Why do you get floating toe with the Weil procedure?	Shortening of MT leads to reduced tension in flexors and PF
How to prevent floating toe?	Pin MTPJ to keep flexor tendon in tension
Diagnostic appearance of a POSITIVE arthrogram for plantar plate tear	Dorsal injection results in leak into FLEXOR sheath
Tailors bunion etiology?	Congenital bowing, **FF splay, incomplete development of DTMTL, mal-insertion of adductor hallucis**, OVERPRONATION
Tailors bunion surgical procedures?	Reverse Hohman, Wilson, Austin, **LODO** (long oblique distal osteotomy)
Types of capsulotomies for 1st MTPJ	**Linear, Inverted L, medial T, H** (transverse plane) **Washington monument**-tightens plantar capsule (STRONGEST) **Mediovertical**-resects PLANTAR capsule
Name 3 types of RA surgical procedures (3)	1) Hoffman-pan MT head resection 2) Hoffman Clayton-pan MT head resection + resection of base of MT 3) Scarf + Weil-joint preserving
Maximum one-step bone graft size to lengthen a brachymetatarsia?	1.5cm if >1.5cm, gradual lengthening
Types of arthropathies?	**seronegative**-reiters/reactive, ankylosing spondylitis, psoriatic **seropositive**-RA, SLE **posttraumatic** **crystal**-gout, CPPD, rheumatoid, septic
Dermatological lesion found in Reiter's disease?	keratoderma blennorrhagicum
What is pannus?	synovial expansion of macrophage, osteoclasts, fibroblast, lymphocytes that destroy cartilage
Chronic gout medical treatment?	allopurinol, probenecid
Acute gout medical treatment?	colchicine, indomethacin
When diagnosing gout, what do uric acid test results indicate?	high-overproducer low-underexcretor

For hammertoe correction surgery, what is the sequence of joints to target?	PIPJ, MTPJ, PIPJ arthrodesis
Hammertoe sequence of release at PIPJ	Tendon, capsule, collateral, arthroplasty
Hammertoe sequence of release at MTPJ	Hood, tendon, capsule, plantar plate
Sequential MTPJ release for hammertoe	arthroplasty, extensor tenotomy, extensor hood, extensor lengthening, flexor to extensor transfer, arthrodesis, MTPJ capsule release, plantar plate release
Ways to describe joint apposition?	congruous, deviated, subluxed/dislocated Depends on the intersection of tangential lines at the articular surfaces
Allopurinol mechanism of action	xanthine oxidase inhibitor
What is xanthine oxidase	enzyme to breakdown purines into uric acid
Probenecid MOA	prevents reabosorption of uric acid @ proximal tubule
How many WBC in a synovial aspirate of septic joint?	>50k
What is Sjogrens' syndrome?	inflammatory disorder of exocrine glands
Blood test for RA	Anti CCP most sensitive
What is dermatomyositis/polymyositis	Symmetrical weakness of limb girdles
What is scleroderma?	CREST: calcinosis, Raynaud's, esophageal dysfunction, sclerodactyly, telangiectasia Induration/thickening/tightening of skin
What is a positive lachman stress test?	>2mm displacement
Uric acid goal in gout	<6 mg/dL
What is the Lepird procedure?	transverse base MT ostoetomy 2-4 for MAA
Location of a Heberden vs Bouchard node?	heberden-DIPJ, bouchard: PIPJ
How many degrees are the angles in Z-plasty?	60
What to rule out for any acute monoarticular arthritis	septic arthritis
What are the types of FDL tendon transfers for treatment of predislocation syndrome?	**Girdlestone Taylor**-original name **Kuwada/Dockery**-reroute thru distal drill hole **Schuberth**-reroute thru proximal drill hole
What defines a skewfoot?	Metatarsus adductus + RF valgus
Difference between heloma molle vs heloma durum?	heloma molle-interdigital due to abutting of condyles

	heloma durum- dorsal IPJ
How often does metatarsus adductus correct itself?	90% self correct in 3 months
What is Heyman Herndon Strong (HHS) procedure?	for surgical treatment of MT adductus, release all TMT and inter cuneiform ligaments except lateral ligaments
Most common location for stress fracture?	2nd MT neck
What stimulates osteophyte production?	loss of functional cartilage
Genetic causes for brachymetatarsia?	Turner's, downs, polio, hyper PTH
3 etiologies for hammertoe?	Flexor Stabilization Extensor Substitution-cavus, weak ant. mm Flexor substitution-weak post. mm
What direction to fuse 1st MTPJ	10 deg valgus/abducted, 10-15 deg DF
Describe the difference between Reverdin vs Reverdin Green vs Reverdin Laird	**Reverdin**-preserve lateral cortex **Green**-preserve sesamoid **Laird**-through lateral cortex, IMA
Name the diagnostic test for diagnosing ankylosing spondylitis	**Schoeber's test**-ability of pt to flex lower back
What is the shape of spine found in patients with ankylosing spondylitis?	kyphosis, also known as poker spine-stiff, inflexible
Name the XR finding for ankylosing spondylitis	Bamboo spine
Name 2 triggers of Reiter syndrome	**STD**-chalymdia, males, URETHRITIS **GI/dysenteric**-shigella, females, children, salmonella, XXXersinia, campylobacter, ENTERITIS (diarrhea)
What is another name for Reiter syndrome?	reactive arthritis
For psoriatic arthritis: List some XR and clinical findings	pencil in cup, whittling HLA-B27, oily pitting nail **salmon pink** papule
Hematogenous spread of septic arthritis is not possible in which age group?	childhood 2-16(vv don't penetrate growth plate)
Which microbe most common in septic joint for children vs IVDU	children-staph aureus, H influenza IVDU-gram negatives
What is the most common viral arthritis	hepatitis B
Which is the MC joint for septic joint	knee
What is the most common fungal arthritis	sporothrix schenckii

What is the name of the rash found in Lyme disease?	Erythema chronicum migrans (bull's eye rash)
What is the name of the pathogen and tick responsible for Lyme disease?	borrelia burgdorferi, deer tick (Ixodes)
Describe the interpretations of straw vs yellow joint fluid color	Straw: non inflammatory arthropathy Yellow: inflammatory High viscosity-normal, non inflammatory Low viscosity-inflammatory
In the diagnosis of gout, is needle birefringement positive or negative?	negative
Is renal or metabolic gout more common?	renal gout (underexcretor)
MC joint affected by pseudogout, XR findings?	knee, Ca2+ deposits in meniscus, cartilage
What is the pseudogout crystal shape? Affects which joint in the foot?	rhomboid, lisfranc
Describe SLE clinical findings, laboratory diagnosis, and treatment	black females with butterfly rash dx with ANA test tx with ANTI MALARIALS
What is scleroderma?	systemic disorder of **connective tissue,** also fibrosis of organs
Describe symptoms of dermatomyositis/polymyositis	**polymyositis**: weakness of limb girdles, **dermatomyositis**: Gottron's papules: flat papules over dorsal knuckles **both have**: heliotrope rash (pink purple) facial lesions
Describe symptoms of Sjogren's syndrome	decreased secretion of exocrine gland, ENLARGED parotid keratoconjunctivitis sicca-dry eyes xerostomia-dry mouth
Describe the clinical test to diagnose Sjogren's syndrome	Schirmer's test-litmus to eye, positive test if <5mm
Describe risk factors for hemarthrosis	bleeding into joint space, risk in hemophilia and pts on warfarin, located at knee/elbow/ankle
What is Baker's cyst?	GANGLION CYST popliteal fossa
What are some early vs late XR findings for RA?	medial erosion except 5th MT EARLY jt space **widening**, LATE jt space **narrowing** (ankylosis)
Name some symptoms found with juvenile RA	skin rash, fever, fusion of C2-C4

What is Still's disease	juvenile RA with a systemic manifestation (splenomegaly, adenopathy)
Describe Churg Strauss sydrome	Small and medium vv vasculitis Arthritis with allergic granulomatosis
Describe Henoch Schnolen purpura	Vasculitis, palpable purpura in LE, arthralgia
What is the normal range for inter-metatarsal angle?	8-12 degrees in rectus foot
what is the Wilson bunionectomy?	Oblique cut to shorten/lateral displace head
What is the Peabody bunionectomy?	Essentially a Reverdin at MT neck
What is the Hohmann bunionectomy?	Essentially a Reverdin Todd at MT neck
What do the Reverdins correct (Reverdin, Green modification, Laird modification, Todd modification)	**Reverdin**-PASA **Green**-PASA **Laird**-PASA/IM **Todd**-PASA, IM, PF MT head
What is the DRATO bunionectomy?	Derotational angulational translational osteotomy MT head can be manipulated at any angle in any plane, unstable
How is the axis guide oriented when performing closing base wedge osteotomies?	**Sagittal plane:** orient perpendicular to WB surface 1. Perpendicular to MT shaft (aim proximally) will DF 2. Aiming distally would PF **Frontal plane:** orient perpendicular to WB surface 1. Aim medially would DF 2. Aim laterally would PF
What is a Logroscino bunionectomy and what is its use?	Reverdin + CBWO Only procedure to correct PASA AND IMA
What is the angle of the chevron osteotomy in a Kalish bunionectomy?	55 degrees
How can troughing from a scarf procedure be fixed?	Apply bone graft in medial intramedullary canal
What is the Lambrinudi procedure used for?	For metatarsus primus elevatus, oblique cut at shaft
What is the difference between the Valenti and Vogler procedure?	**Valenti**: joint destructive, dorsal portions of prox phalanx and 1st MT head removed **Vogler**: offset V osteotomy apex at metaphyseal diaphyseal jcn, long dorsal arm, 40 deg cut
What is a Regnauld procedure	Peg in hole (mexican hat)
What is the purpose of a mediovertical capsulotomy?	Resect redundant plantar capsule

Which capsulotomy tightens the medial capsule?	Washington monument
Describe the stages of the Drago Orloff Jacobs classification	1) pain end ROM (FUNCTIONAL) 2) limited ROM, flat MT head (ADAPTATION) 3) pain full ROM (REMODELING) 4) fusion <10 deg ROM (LIMITATION)
List all the treatments for hallux varus	1) soft tissue release 1st MTPJ 2) med capsulotomy 3) tibial sesamoidectomy 4) EHL transfer to plantarlat prox phalanx 5) Jt destructive 6) Fusion

Pes Planus & Associated Conditions

QUESTION	ANSWER
Procedures to correct flatfoot in transverse plane?	Evans, calcaneal cuboid distraction arthrodesis (CCDA), med cuneiform closing wedge osteotomy
Purpose of adding Lapidus or Cotton procedure to Evans?	Stability of the first ray will PF the first ray and help the PL exert its action more proximally
Side effects of an arthroeresis? Indications?	Talar fracture, migration Good as an ADJUNCT Impact blocking-prevents anterior displacement of lateral talar process
Congenital vs acquired flatfoot	**Congenital**: tarsal coalition, CVT, talipes calcaneovalgus (TCV), KIDNER foot **Acquired**: PTTD
Discussion of ORIF vs fusion for Lisfranc fracture?	Studies by COETZEE and HENNING showed that a lot of ORIF resulted in 1) arthritis 2) hardware removal 3) conversion to fusion Surgery necessary to assess amount of soft tissue interposition and high likelihood of cartilaginous comminution
Procedures to correct flatfoot in sagittal plane?	**Cotton** **Young**-reroute TA through navicular with insertion intact **Cobb**-split TA , graft reroute through medial cuneiform, tenodese with PTT
Johnson and Strom Classification 2A vs 2B?	2A <30% TN uncovering 2B >30% TN uncovering

What is the Cobb procedure?	Proximal split TA reroute thru medial cuneiform→ tenodesed to PTT Used for PTTD
What is the Lowman procedure?	TN fusion + TA rerouted through navicular→ tenodesed to spring ligament
How to orient cut for a medial calcaneal slide osteotomy?	Dorsal posterior→plantar anterior
Where to perform osteotomy in Evans procedure? Size of graft?	1.5cm prox to CCJ 1cm graft
Classification system for PT tendon MRI in PTTD	Conti
Classification for location of PT rupture in PTTD	Funk
Function of spring ligament?	support talar head, medial arch stabilization
Where to insert Evans graft? Why?	1.3cm proximal to CC to avoid anterior facet
How does Evans procedure work biomechanically?	adducting the foot increases the lever arm for the PL and windlass mechanism to recreate arch
What is the Miller procedure?	NC and FMCJ fusion
What is Lowman procedure?	TN fusion + TA rerouted under navicular, attached to spring ligament
Accessory navicular classification, which ones most common	1-os tibiale externum 2-synchondrosis A-parallel, B-plantar 3-gorilloid navicular types 2 and 3 make 70%
What does arthroeresis mean?	limitation of joint movement
How does an arthroeresis work?	prevents the lateral facet of talus from hitting the floor of sinus tarsi
What angles are DECREASED in pes planus	CIA (obviously), 1st MT declination, FF adductus
Types of arthroeresis?	impact blocking, axis alterting, self locking

Pes Cavus

QUESTION	ANSWER
Describe the Jones tenosuspension procedure	transfer EHL to 1st MT head, fuse distal stump to EHB. fuse hallux IPJ

Describe the Hibbs tenosuspension procedure	EDL tendon strips transferred to lateral cuneiform, EDL stumps fused to EDB, digital fusions
What is the split tibialis anterior tendon transfer? (STATT)	Tibialis anterior tendon split from insertion until proximal to superior extensor retinaculum. 1/2 of TA to cuboid or peroneus tertius
What is the Heyman procedure?	transfer EDL to MT neck
Where is the tibialis anterior tendon transferred for cavus correction?	lateral cuneiform
What is the Hoke procedure?	NC(1 and 2) plantar based CBWO, arthrodesis
What are the 3 types of anterior cavus?	metatarsus cavus-TMT lesser tarsus-NC, forefoot cavus-chopart jt
What is cut in Steindler stripping?	LPL, plantar fascia, first layer of plantar muscles (abductor hallucis, abductor digiti minimi, FDB)
What is the Cole procedure?	CBWO at NCJ
What is Kirby's sign?	posterior facet abuts floor of calcaneus to occlude sinus tarsi, sign of maximum pronation
3 types of cavus?	Metatarsus, lesser tarsus, forefoot

Ankle Pathology

QUESTION	ANSWER
Positive anterior drawer test? Positive talar tilt test?	>1cm or >3-8mm compared to contralateral side >4-5 deg compared to contralateral side
Do you lag a syndesmostic screw?	No, you do not want to compress ankle joint
Ankle sprain classification?	O' Donoghue (partial, partial + function loss, complete) Leach 1) ATFL, 2) ATFL + CFL 3) ATFL + CFL + PTFL Dias
Radiographic measurement to assess for fibular shortening?	Tibiotalar ligament 8-15 degrees or <83 degrees
MC Lauge Hansen ankle fracture pattern	SER2
What does Lauge Hansen classification describe?	First word-position of FOOT relative to ground Second word-position of TALUS relative to ground

Describe a Lauge Hansen PAB 1, 2, 3 pattern	1-Transverse med mall 2-AITFL or PITFL 3-Lateral spike or butterfly lateral mall
Based on Lauge Hansen, when is the only time you can get LCL rupture?	SAD1
Based on Lauge Hansen, when is the only time you CAN'T get MCL rupture?	SAD2
What is it called when the PTT is interposed in medial malleolus?	Coonrad bugg trap
How would you close reduce an ankle?	1) sedate the patient OR do hematoma block: 20 gauge needle medial to TAT at ankle joint. Aspirate hematoma then inject 12cc 1% lido PLAIN
Indications for ankle surgery (2)?	1. UNABLE TO CLOSE REDUCE: displacement >2mm or >15 deg angulation 2. Unstable ankle--2 breaks in the ring (2/3 including medial mall, lateral mall, or posterior mall)
When would interfragmentary screw alone be sufficient without need for neutralization plate?	1. no comminution 2. long oblique fx's
Concerns for a diabetic with ankle fracture?	Technically none unless >1 comorbidity 1) Charcot 2) locking plate 3) prolonged NWB AT LEAST 3 MONTHS (poor bone healing) 4) poor wound healing/infection, for those with NEUROPATHY, DOUBLE the fixation (WUKICH) TREAT AS CHARCOT STAGE 1
1) Do you need to fix syndesmosis with bi-malleolar fixation? 2) What about if posterior mall fixed?	1) NO (YAMAGUCHI) stated that enough soft tissue to hold syndesmosis together 2) No need if posterior mall fixed also
What is the "Boden criteria" (1989) in regards to guidelines for syndesmotic fixation?	Fixate only if fracture >4.5cm proximal from distal tip (longer lever arm more unstable)
How to treat OCD of ankle fracture?	**SMALL lesions**: Arthroscopy-remove fracture debris and penetrate bone to stimulate bleeding **LARGE lesions**: OATS, talar en block (for OATS failure)
What type of irrigation is best for ankle arthroscopy?	Lactated ringers better than normal saline because better chondrocyte metabolism
What is Bassett's ligament?	**Thickened** accessory AITFL, can cause ANTEROLATERAL ankle impingement, synovitis, s/p inversion injury

What is a Dupuytrens fracture?	Bi mall (same as Potts)
Which is the deepest portion of the deltoid ligament?	Anterior tibiotalar
When is CT for ankle needed?	Comminution, unable to assess degree of posterior mall involvement
Which article set the foundation for the importance of bringing the fibula out to length when performing an ORIF of an ankle fracture?	**Yablon** in JBJS stated that the talus follows the fibula, so reducing the fibula and bringing it out to length would act as a butress for the fibula
Why is it important to perform surgery on an unstable ankle fracture?	**Ramsey** in JBJS stated that a 1mm lateral displacement of the talus would lead to 42% decrease in ankle articulation.
What are 2 ways of fixing the syndesmosis in an ankle?	1) Tightrope (Arthrex ® because it maintains motion at syndesmosis, lower rates of malreduction, earlier WB, no need for hardware removal 2) 2 x 4.5 screws (3.5 is okay) each purchasing 3 cortices. 4.5 screws are easier to remove
What is the proper orientation to insert a syndesmotic screw? How many degrees relative to coronal plane?	posterolateral fibula—>anteromedial tibia 25 deg relative to coronal plane
What is a Bosworth fracture?	fibular fracture from PITFL
What is a Volkmann fracture?	posterior mall fracture, from PITFL
When is it appropriate to remove a syndesmotic screw?	12 wks
What is the proper position of foot while inserting syndesmotic screw screw?	Dorsiflexion because talar dome wider ANTERIORLY
When is it appropriate to perform arthrogram for ankle sprain?	Acutely, after 5-7 days fibrosis seal off injury
MC nerve injury ankle sprain?	Peroneal N
What is the normal angle between ATFL and CFL? What is the use of this angle?	132 degrees useful for stress XR, arthrography, MRI axis
Describe the Essex lopresti classification for calcaneal fractures	A-tongue type, B-joint depression
Osteochondral autograft transplant system (OATS) procedure vs talar en block procedure?	Osteochondral autograft transplant system (OATS): cylinder of cartilage from NWB surface transferred to area of defect Talar en block-wedge from allograft

Clinical presentation for OCD?	Ankle "locking" pain 8wk s/p ankle sprain
Comminuted fibula is a Lauge Hansen___? What is a good hardware to use for a comminuted fibula?	PAB 3, bridging plate
What is a Berndt Harty 1?	Subchondral fx of the talar dome
What is a common sport that causes peroneal subluxation?	Skiing
2 types of ankle brace?	Stirrup (air cast) Lace-up (Arizona brace)
How long to be in ankle brace, then what?	2 wks, then elastic compression WBAT
Trimalleolar fracture also known as?	Cotton
Bi-malleolar fx also known as?	Pott's fracture
Tri-planar fx also known as?	Salter 2 or 3
Ankle arthroscopy port locations?	Anteromedial, anterolateral
Name of meedial malleolar fracture classification system	Mueller
What did the Ramsey article state?	1mm lateral displacement of talus = 42% decrease in ankle articulation
What to do if you only find a posterior mall and med mall fracture on XR?	get XR higher up leg, probably have a PER 4
What is a Blair fusion procedure for the ankle?	Remove talar BODY + tibial graft into talar neck
What is a Volkmann fracture? When is it appropriate to fixate these fractures?	posterior malleolus, when involves >25% joint
In the screw fixation of distal fibula, how many cortices are crossed?	one distal to fracture line (prevent entering into ankle joint) two proximal to fracture line
What is the ligament of Lazaro?	**fibulotalocalcaneal ligament**
How do you splint the ankle after closed reduction?	HEAVILY PADDED, Jones compression splint WAWA (webril ACE, Webril ACE)
What are the 4 ligaments of distal tibial fibular syndesmosis? Which ligament is the strongest?	AITFL, PITFL, inferior transverse lig, interosseus lig (PITFL strongest 35%, followed by AITFL 33%)

What are the parts of deltoid ligament?	Superficial-tibiocalcaneal (strongest), talonavicular, superficial **posterior** tibiotalar Deep-ant tibiotalar, deep posterior tibiotalar other: fibers to spring ligament, posterior to spring ligament, deep talocalcaneal
What are the functions of superficial and deep deltoid ligament?	superficial-prevent eversion deep-prevent axial rotation
Which OCD fragment is described as "deep cup" vs "shallow wafer"?	deep cup-media (PIMP) shallow wafer-lateral (DIAL)
What is the vassal phenomenon?	correction of the primary deformity will allow others to correct
Which nerve can be injured at the anterolateral port in ankle arthroscopy?	superficial peroneal, visualize by flexing 4th toe
Which position does the Quigley maneuver put foot into?	supinated, adducted, internal rotaiton
Describe the Charnley technique for closed reduction	Exaggerate, distract, and reverse Pressure at site, proximal/distal to fracture
When is an ankle fracture an emergency?	when talus cannot be reduced
What is a butterfly fragment, what is the mechanism to cause this type of pattern?	in ankle fracture (PAB) wedge of long bone created by two oblique fracture lines from a compressive bending force and a distracting force
What type of hardware is needed to fixate a distal lateral malleolar fracture?	2.7 interfrag screw, 1/3 tubular plate. want 6 cortices proximal to fracture, 4 distal
Is complete rupture of syndesmotic complex a necessary for Maisonneuve fracture? Is ORIF needed to repair a Maisonneuve fracture?	NO, NO
How many cortices do syndesmotic screws need to purchase?	tri or quadracortical 1 across 4 or can use 2 screws
What is a Brostrom procedure?	anatomical repair of lateral ligaments with imbrication
What are some "non anatomical" repair of ankle ligaments?	**Evans**-PB thru fibula ant—>post **Watson Jones**-PB thru fibula post —> ant repair ATFL **Chrisman Snook**-split PB
What is the classification system for peroneal subluxation?	**Eckert and Davis** 1-retinaculum separates from fibrocartilage (Most common) 2-fibrocartilaginous ridge detaches from fibula

	3-fibular avulsion fracture
What are some eponyms for for bimalleolar fractures?	Pott's or Dupuytren
Is a transsyndesmotic screw a lag screw?	no, it is only for reducing the ankle joint, you dont want to compress the ankle gutters.

Achilles & Rearfoot Pathology

QUESTION	ANSWER
What percent of calcaneal fractures lead to compartment syndrome	15-20%
% of STJ ROM after TN fusion?	8%
Degree of ROM in remaining joints after TN fusion?	2 degrees
Normal amount of TN ROM (in degrees)?	37 degrees
Side effect of endoscopic plantar fasciotomy?	lateral column instability leading to CCJ impingement
How to perform triple arthrodesis?	resect MTJ then STJ fuse STJ then MTJ
Treatment for middle facet talocalcaneal coalition?	Resect, insert adipose tissue, or any kind of soft tissue
What are some etiologies of plantar fasciitis?	Equinus or hamstring tightness (increased load on FF and windlass), overpronation, obesity, fat pad atrophy, DISH/acromegaly
In a plantar fasciotomy, what is released?	Baxter's nerve, remove MEDIAL 1/3-1/2 of plantar fascia
What is Hoffa's sign?	Less taut Achilles tendon
What are some physical exam and radiographic sequalelae of tarsal coalition?	Peroneal spastic flatfoot, ball and socket ankle joint, equinus, arthrosis of adjacent joints, calcaneofib remodeling
How many degrees left in STJ after TN fusion?	2 deg ROM in remaining jts OR 8% left in STJ ASTION
Achilles rupture risk factors	Overuse, biomechanical (planus/cavus), old age, improper training (weekend warrior), fluoroquinolones, steroids

	MOSTLY MIDSUBSTANCE
How to perform Thompson test?	With patient prone, knee bent, in ruptured Achilles, find a loss of ankle PF
Where to make incision for surgical repair of Achilles?	MEDIAL to tendon
Rerupture rate for conservative treatment of Achilles rupture?	VARIES, 20% for conservative, 5% for surgical
What can be used for interposition after a resection of a coalition?	BONE WAX, EDB, adipose
What are some Achilles lengthening procedures to perform in chronic Achilles rupture?	**Bugg and Boyd** (3 strips fascia lata), **Bosworth**-strip of gastroc aponeurosis, peroneus brevis T, FHL, plantaris
What are the borders of Kager's triangle?	Achilles, FHL, superior calc
What are the side effects of STJ fusion?	lose mobile adaptor, lose shock absorption, arthritis at ankle, MTJ,
Order of joints to fuse in a triple arthrodesis? Which joint has highest nonunion rates? Which joint is the most important to fuse?	TN→TC→CC TN highest nonunion rates TN most important
What is the magic angle effect?	structures angled at 55 degrees in MRI appear hyper intense
What is the paratenon?	loose connective tissue sheath over tendon
Where does peroneus quartus insert?	peroneal tubercle
What is the most common complication for surgical repair of Achilles tendon?	wound dehiscence (15%)
At what point along the leg does the sural nerve cross the Achilles?	9.83cm proximal to insertion
What are some reasons to perform a medial incision when repairing the Achilles?	prevent adhesions, prevent wound dehiscence, avoid sural N, lesser saph
What are 2 mechanisms for Achilles rupture?	landing on PF foot, violent PF with foot planted
Where is the Achilles watershed area located?	2-6cm proximal to insertion
What are the risks of Achilles re-rupture?	18% conservative, 2% surgical (some other studies shown to be the same)
Which compartment of the leg do you find peroneal artery?	posterior, not lateral compartment
What does plantar fascia attach to distally?	plantar plate

What is the clinical triad for presentation of tarsal coalition?	pain, limitation ROM, muscle spasm
What are the ages of ossification for tarsal coalitions?	TN (3-5) CN (8-12) TC (12-15)
What is the Murphy procedure?	transfer Achilles insertion to dorsal calcaneus to weaken lever arm (dec PF 50%) for tx cerebral palsy
What is the Cowell/Badgley procedure?	CN bar excision with interposition of EDB
What is injured in sinus tarsi syndrome?	interosseus talocalcaneal ligament
What are the 3 phases of tendon healing	inflammatory, proliferative, maturation
What is the triad of clinical presentation for Haglund's disease?	postero LATERAL calc, AITC, bursitis
What is Mattle's test?	Excess DF with pt prone, knee bent
What is Simmond's test?	XS DF with pt prone, knee NOT bent
Which coalition is typically the most symptomatic	CN
What are 3 surgical procedure Haglund's deformity?	Keck and Kelly-dorsal CWO Duvries-bumpectomy with LATERAL approach Fowler and Philip-bumpectomy with POSTERIOR approach, mercedes (inverted Y incision)
Where is the incision made for a medial approach for triple arthrodesis?	Med malleolus to NCJ
What is the order of resection and fixation of the joints in triple arthrodesis?	**Resection**: MTJ (CC TN) then STJ **Fixation**: STJ then MTJ (TN, CC)
List the 3 types of arthroeresis	**Insert laterally distal to POSTERIOR FACET** 1) **Self locking wedge**-prevent lat talus from hitting floor calc (MBA) 2) **Impact blocking (stem)**-prevent ant displacement of lat talus (STA peg) 3) **Axis altering**-ramp to elevate floor sinus tarsi (Sgarlato mushroom)
For ankle arthroscopy: 1. Where is the anterocentral port inserted? 2. Where is the anterolateral port inserted? 3. What is the MOST COMMON INJURED N IN ANKLE ARTHROSCOPY?	1. **Anterocentral**: between EHL and EDL tendons, avoid ant tib A and **deep peron N** 2. **Anterolateral**: lateral to peroneus tertius and medial to lateral mall 3. MC injured NERVE: superficial peroneal (intermediate dorsal cutaneous)

Question	Answer
What are the steps in repair of pilon fractures?	1) Reduce fibula 2) Realign articular surface of tibia 3) Apply bone graft as necessary 4) Apply buttress plate
What is a Blair fusion?	Salvage when talar body missing or can't be salvaged. Tibial graft into talar head
What is dynamization?	All wires/pins loosened pt allowed to WB. Allows for axial forces without distraction to strengthen bone
What is ligamentotaxis?	Pull fracture fragments into alignment using distraction
What are the advantages of external fixation?	Decreases soft tissue dissection, infection, early ROM/WB, post op angular adjustment
How is the amount of callus distraction calculated?	Compress x 7 days 1mm per day MAXIMUM wait 2x amount of distraction time
Where are the incisions made in a fasciotomy for treatment of compartment syndrome of the foot?	Over 2nd interspace and 4th interspace
Name 2 physical exam tests to evaluate for syndesmotic injury	Distal and proximal leg compression, external rotation test
How is it determined if a coalition should be fused or resected?	Fuse if >50% of joint involved

Trauma

QUESTION	ANSWER
What is the Rosenthal nail trauma classification system?	**Rosenthal**-1) distal to phalanx 2) distal lunula 3) proximal lunula
Most common digital fracture	5th digit, also known as "bedpost fracture"
What is the proper position to fuse hindfoot?	0-5 degrees valgus, relative to the ground. Use the floor of sinus tarsi and lateral talar process 2-4 deg of calc eversion during stance is necessary "THOU SHALL NOT VARUS"
How to sedate patient for closed reduction?	IV versed (midazolam) and morphine

What is a nutcracker fracture?	Fracture resulting from compression of cuboid and anterior calcaneal process
Why does a dislocated talar neck fracture require emergent treatment?	Close reduce to preserve blood supply to prevent AVN of talus
What are some weaknesses with IM screw for 5th MT base fixation?	Osteoporosis, avulsion fx (small fragment)
What is the pathophysiology of compartment syndrome?	Interstitial pressure **exceeds capillary hydrostatic pressure** so microcirculation shuts down
When is it appropriate to close soft tissue after an open fracture?	Not until it soft tissue damage has demarcated and is clear it isn't going to necrose
What is the purpose of external fixation for an open fracture?	Reduce and STABILIZE the fracture and hold in place w/o dissection, Compromised soft tissue
XR findings to rule out Lisfranc injury?	**AP**-1st and 2nd MT, 1st and 2nd MT diastasis **MO**-4th MT and cuboid, 3rd MT **LAT**-FMCJ
Other injuries to rule out out after calcaneal fracture?	1) L1 fracture 2) pelvic fx 3) urethral trauma
Most common deformed position of calcaneus after fracture?	VARUS
What are some good indications for non-operative treatment of calcaneal fracture? Negative consequences?	Nondisplaced Severe PAD, DM Elderly household ambulators **However,** some studies say 5.5x MORE likely → arthrodesis for arthritis. Regardless, conversion to arthrodesis rates after ORIF are high as well
Stewart classification	E-jones I-intra at base E-avulsion I-comminuted O-apophysis
List the 4 surgical goals for ORIF of the calcaneus	Maintain height, width, length, articular surface
When is an open fracture considered contaminated vs infected	An open fracture is **contaminated** unless it is left open without treatment for 6-8 hrs when it becomes **infected**
What is a Greenstick fracture?	Incomplete fracture involving only one cortex
What is the risk of removing both sesamoids in 1st MTPJ trauma surgery?	Hallux malleus
Which stage in the Jahss classification is surgery indicated?	1A-conjoined ligament prevents closed reduction, deformity too tight
What are the percentage risk of AVN in the stages of the	1-10%,

Hawkin's classification	2-40%, 3-90% 4-100%
Describe the Ruedi Allgower classification system	1) Nondisplaced 2) Displacement 3) Displacement + comminution
What is the location watershed zone of the posterior tibial tendon?	Behind med mall
What is the location watershed zone of the tibialis anterior tendon?	1-2cm from insertion
What bacteria is associated with cat scratch fever	Bartonella henslae
Which part of the navicular is LEAST vascular?	Central 1/3
Describe the outcomes between operative vs nonoperative treatment for displaced intraarticular calcaneal fractures	Same (Buckley et al, JBJS), however ORIF makes it easier to convert to STJ fusion in the future
What is the mechanism of injury for a lateral talar process fracture?	Dorsiflexion INVERSION (AKA snowboarder's fracture)
List important clinical information to gather after a patient sustains an ankle fracture	Neurovascular status, open wounds? Tetanus status? Blisters? Headache, dizziness, blurry vision, chest pain, difficulty breathing, NPO status
Describe 3 locations to make incisions in ORIF For Lisfranc fracture/dislocation	1) medial to 1st 2) 2nd interspace 3) 4th interspace
Describe the mechanism of injury of shepard's fracture of the talus	forced PF with compression of posterior process between tibia and calcaneus
What is a "sand toe" injury?	opposite of turf toe, it is the hyper-flexion
In calcaneal fractures, which fragment is described as "thalamic or comet" and which is "semilunar"	lateral fragment in calcaneal fractures essex lopresti A tongue type- thalamic/comet essex lopresti B- semilunar
In compartment syndrome, how soon does a fasciotomy need to be performed?	8 hrs is when nerve damage, 3 hours muscle damage
Describe the mechanism of injury in Lisfranc injuries	twisting on axially loaded foot, usually dorsal dislocation
List the radiographic angles used to measure 5th MT pathology	IMA Fallat and Buckholz-4th MT and medial cortex of 5th LDA-5th MT and medial cortex of 5th

List the 3 surgical goals for ORIF of ankle fractures	1) fibular height 2) ankle mortise 3) syndesmosis
Describe the difference between Quenu and Kuss vs Hardcastle classification	Quenu and Kuss: homolateral, isolated, divergent Hardcastle: total, partial, divergent
Describe the classification system for navicular fractures	Watson Jones 1-tuberosity 2-dorsal avulsion 3A-coronal 3B-major medial fragment 3C-comminution of lateral 4-stress fracture
Describe the Jahss classification	1-dislocation 2A- + intersesamoid ligament rupture 2B- + sesamoid fracture 2C- + conjoined ligament tear
Describe the Torg classification system	1-acute jones 2-delayed union (6 mo), IM sclerosis 3-nonunion (9 mo) fx widening, IM sclerosis canal obliteration
Describe the Lawrence and Bott classification	1-avulsion, 2-jones, 3-diaphysis
List the 6 P's of compartment syndrome	pain, parasthesia paresis, pallor, pulselessness, paralysis,
Describe the Sneppen classification	1-OCD (compression) 2-body (shear) 3-posterior 4-lateral 5-crush
Which fragment is "constant fragment" in calcaneal fracture?	fragment under sustentaculum tali due to deltoid ligament (question as to if it is truly constant)
What is another name for Cedell's fracture?	posteromedial process of talus
What is another name for Shepard's fracture	posterolateral process of talus
How is compartment syndrome diagnosed?	> 30mmhg or 10-30mmHg less than diastolic BP
What is the name of calcaneal piece attached to Achilles from calcaneal fracture?	tuber
List 2 reasons you need to ORIF a MT shaft fracture	1) displacement > 2mm, 2) >10deg angulation
What is Boden's criteria in regards to the fixation of	fix syndesmosis ONLY if deltoid injury AND

syndesmosis?	>4.5cm proximal extension of fibular fx
Describe the Hardcastle classification	A-homolateral B-partial (1st medial OR 2-4 lateral) C-divergent (1st medial AND 2-4 lateral)
List the antibiotics involved in the Gustillo Anderson open fracture classification	1: 1st gen cephalosporin (Ancef) 2: ancef + clinda 3: ancef, clinda + aminoglycoside

Pediatric Pathology

QUESTION	ANSWER
What is the treatment for pediatric deformity of tibial torsion?	WATCHFUL WAITING (most resolve by 6 yo) Derotational supra malleolar osteotomy
List some causes of juvenile HAV Which surgical procedures should be avoided?	Atavistic cuneiform, pronation, NM dz, flatfoot Avoid soft tissue procedures 2/2 high recurrence
List the order bones ossify from birth to 4 years	0 year-cuboid (birth) 1 year-lateral cuneiform, 2 year-medial cuneiform, 3 year-intermediate cuneiform, 4 year-navicular
List some medial soft tissues that can be released in treatment of clubfoot deformity	Posterior tibial tendon Z plasty, superficial deltoid, TN ligament
List some contraindications for arthroeresis	Internal femoral torsion, knee angular deformity, peroneal spasm, ligamentous laxity
Tillaux fractures are more common in which patient age group?	More common in adolescents (medial growth plate has began to fuse). Usually due to SER injury, categorized as Salter Harris 3
What is a triplane fracture?	Salter Harris 2-4--anterior epiphyseal fracture with posteromedial metaphyseal fragment
What is Salter Harris 5, 6, 7	5-compression-injury to epiphysis 6-peripheral physis, angular deformity 7-epiphysis avulsion
What is Clarks' rule for pediatric dosing?	Child's weight x adult dose / 150
What is the Thurston Holland sign? Describe the Salter Harris classification system for pediatric fractures	**metaphyseal spike from salter harris 2** 1-through growth plate 2-above

	3-below 4-both 5-crush 6-missing epiphysis
What is a Talipes calcaneus?	a DF'ed calcaneus resulting in calcaneal gait
What is congenital curly toe known as?	clinodactyly
Which Salter Harris fracture pattern is the MC?	2 (Thurston Holland sign)
For a Ganley splint, where is the torque bar positioned for either an internal or external rotation deformity?	**internal rotation deformity**: rearfoot **external rotation deformity**: forefoot
What is the use of a Denis Browne bar?	Clubfoot or MAA, flatfoot, riveted on shoe
Name the 4 types of congenital flatfoot	1) CVT, RIGID! 2) Talipes calcaneovalgus (TCV) (flexible pes planovalgus) 3) Tarsal coalition (RIGID) 4) Kidner foot
What is a Fillauer bar?	Denis Browne with clamps to shoe
What is a unibar?	Denis Browne bar with ball and socket joint which can be tightened to varus position
What is a counter rotation system (LANGER)?	AKA Langer, Denis Browne with HINGES for better tolerated
What is a Bebax shoe?	treats MT adductus after casting (FF to RF abnormalities)
What is a Wheaton brace?	AFO with medial flare alternative for casting MAA,
What is a Wheaton brace system, and its use?	AFO above and below knee to keep knee 90 deg prevent femur/hip twisting to tx TIBIAL TORSION
What are twister cables used for?	tx scissors gait in CP pts belt around waist to control abduction at heel contact,
What is a Friedman counter splint?	belt around posterior heel
Describe the components that make up APGAR, what is the normal range?	normal 8-10 appearance, pulse, grimace, activity, resp effort

Describe the developmental landmarks from age 3months to 3 years	3mo-lift head 6mo-roll over 9-mo-sit up 12mo-stand 14-walk 15-18-words 18-21combine words 21-24 3 word sentence 3 yr propulsive gait
What is the cause of Blount's cadisease in infants vs adults	**infants**-early walking & obesity **adults**-trauma/infection can lead to BOWING
At what age does Kohler's disease appear?	3-6
What are some causes for congenitally dislocated hip?	breech, oligohydramnios, first born
What does the Ortolani maneuver do?	Relocates hip, a physical exam for congenitally dislocated hip
What does the Barlow maneuver do?	Dislocates hip, a physical exam for congenitally dislocated hip
What is known as Anchor's sign?	butt cheek wrinkles on dislocated hip
What is known as Galleazi's (Allis sign)	one knee higher than other when flexed
What are 2 etiologies of clubfoot?	**AKA talipes equinovarus (TEV)** **1) Idiopathic**-(intrauterine-first born, breech) **2) acquired**-NM disorder-arthrogryphosis, CP, spina bifida
What is Simon's rule of 15?	1) talo 1st MT angle >15 degrees 2) Kite's angle <15 degrees

Describe congenital vertical talus (CVT):
  1. Is it flexible?
  2. Associated with what systemic disease?
  3. Gait?
  4. Forefoot position?
  5. RF position?
  6. Treatment?
  7. Talus shape?
	AKA Persian slipper, Convex pes planovalgus. Calcaneus rectus or plantarflexed
	  1. RIGID rocker bottom
	  2. **Arthrogryphosis**-multiple joint contractures
	  3. Peg leg gait
	  4. FF ABducted, dorsiflexed
	  5. Calcaneus in valgus, equinus
	  6. CANNOT CAST!!! (rigid deform) Surgery REQUIRED. Soft tissue only for skin stretching
	  7. **HOURGLASS** talar neck

List some surgical procedures for CVT at ages 1-4 yo vs 4-6yo vs >12 yo	1-4 ORIF TNJ 4-6 (Green price procedure: extra articular

	arthrodesis) >12 yo triple arthrodesis
Should a flexible pes planus deformity in infants be a concern?	No, most infants develop arch in 1st decade
List some radiographic findings for talocalcaneal coalition	talar beak, broad lateral talar process, narrow post STJ facet, ball and socket ankle jt
List some symptoms for MT adductus How do they compensate?	TRIPPING, inc risk of 5th MT base fx Compensate by PRONATION
Do all cases of MT adductus in infants need treatment?	86% resolve w/o treatment
List the types of MT adductus	**Dynamic**-born straight, tightening of ABductor hallucis causes C foot **Flexible** **Rigid**
List osseus procedures for treatment of MT adductus	For patients >8yo Lepird, Berman and Gartland (lateral crescentic)
List soft tissue procedures for treatment of MT adductus	**HHS** **Thompson** (abductor hallucis resection)
List all the types of polydactyly. Which one is MC?	distal phalanx duplication **wide head with normal shaft (MC)** T-shaped Y-shaped complete ray duplication well formed vs rudimentary
Macrodactylyl is seen with which medical condition?	Neurofibromatosis Macrodactylyl risks vascular compromise
What is the MC metatarsal affected by brachymetisa	1st or 4th
What is the MC form of cerebral palsy?	spastic due to adductor spasticity
What is the clinical presentation of the musculature of muscular dystrophy patients?	**Pseudohypertrophy**-apparent hypertrophy that is actually fat not mm!
Describe the Duchenne's disease: 1. Age affected? 2. Pathognomic sign 3. IQ? 4. How is it diagnosed? 5. Genetics?	1. 2-5, pulmonary disorder die at age 20 2. Gower's sign, toe walking, waddling gait 3. **low IQ** 4. diagnosed with muscle biopsy 5. sex linked recessive
Describe Becker's disease 1. physical presentation 2. IQ?	1. Mild duchenne, pes cavus, die at 40 2. no IQ drop

What disease would you find "Popeye arms"	Facioscapulohumeral muscular dystrophy
List 3 radiographic findings in clubfoot	1. **Horizontal breech**-bimalleolar axis <75 (hindfoot to malleolar plane) is positive 2. **Beatson and pearson**-AP talocalc + lateral talocalc <40 is positive 3. **Simon's rule** of 15
What is the position of the talar head/neck in CVT?	Adduction and PF
Casting can be used to treat all pediatric conditions EXCEPT?	Clubfoot, MAA, calcaneovalgus, windswept deformity, BUT NOT CVT
What is a risk for treating MT adductus with reverse last shoes?	PRONATION of MTJ and RF can lead to SKEWFOOT
Which foot ligaments are contracted in CVT?	Tibionavicular and Talonavicular
What is ectrodactylyl?	Lobster claw 2/2 teratogen, chromosomal abnormality
What is the MC congenital deformity in the foot?	SYNDACTYLY
What are some physical exam findings for talipes calcaneovalgus (TCV)	FLEXIBLE flatfoot, dorsum of foot touches anterior shin, calcaneus DF
List some risks for clubfoot casting	AVN talar head, DF navicular on calcaneus, valgus (overcorrection), rockerbottom, navicular subluxation (MTJ subluxation)

Radiology & Angles

QUESTION	ANSWER
Which calcaneal XR view can be used to visualize lateral widening and varus deformity?	Calcaneal axial view
In MRI imaging, what is STIR useful in visualizing?	Short tau inversion recovery Fat suppression, high water signal BONE MARROW ABNORMALITIES
What is the MR grading for ankle sprains?	1-partial ligamentous tear 2-partial ligamentous tear+ functional impairment 3-complete ligamentous tear
Which radiographic view is used to view the os calcaneus secundarius? Which radiographic view is used to view the os tibiale	os calcaneus secundarius: MO os tibiale externum: LO

externum?	
Describe x-ray findings for a STJ coalition	talar beaking, broad lateral process of talus, NARROW posterior STJ facet
On MRI, at calcaneal insertion, a normal Achilles appears concave or convex?	concave
Which radiographic angle is most predictive of plantar Charcot ulceration?	Meary's angle >27 or Hibb's angle
How is Bohler's angle measured?	Line connecting points on the calcaneal tuberosity, posterior facet, anterior beak
How is the angle of Gissane measured?	Line connecting points on the posterior facet, anterior shelf
List the phases of a bone scan	1-flow (angiogram) 2-blood pool (hyperemia or ischemia) 3-delayed phase (rate of bone meabolism) 4-diagnosis of OM
What is rarefaction?	decreased density of bone on XR similar to periosteal reaction
How would wood appear on ultrasound	hyperechoic with hypo echoic shadow
What is Hawkin's sign	Radiolucency in bone 2/2 to washout of bone due to good blood supply @ 6-8 wks
Name the 3 structural radiographic angles	IMA, CIA, MAA
Name the positional radiographic angles	HAA, TSP, Meary's, Seiberg's index, 1st MT dec, 5th MT dec
What is the forefoot adductus angle? Normal? What is its effect in pronation/supination?	FF to RF, normal 0-10, slightly less than MAA pron-decrease, supination-increase
What is the lesser tarsus adductus angle? Normal? What is its effect in pronation/supination?	AKA lesser tarsus angle, midfoot to RF, pronation-inc, supination-decrease
How to take calcaneal axial film, what does it view? How to take Harris Beath film, what does it view?	Calc axial: supine, beam at 45, view post calc-calc widening, varus/valgus Harris Beath: calcaneal axial in ski jumper position, view tarsal coalition,
What are some terms used to describe osteomyelitis on XR?	Periosteal reaction, osteolysis, sclerosis, eburnation, loss of cortical margin
What is kVp?	peak kilovoltage the energy of electrons determining the

	maximum voltage across XR tube controls the contrast
What is mAs?	miliampere second, primary controlling factor of radiographic density and photon #
What is the normal 5th IMA?	normal: 6.47 <7 abnormal: 8.71
Which midfoot bone is not present at birth? When does it ossify?	navicular, ossifies 2-5 y.o
What is Kite's angle? What is the normal range? Increased or decreased in pes planus?	AP talocalc, normal 20-40 degrees, increased in planus
What are all the angles seen in lateral view and their normal values? Which 2 decrease in flatfoot?	Calcanal inclination angle (CIA)-24.5 degrees (decreases in flatfoot) talar declination-21 degrees lateral talocalcaneal (CIA + TD)-45 degrees 1st MT declination-19-25 degrees (decreases in flatfoot) Meary's (talo 1st MT)-0 degrees Kirby's sign Cyma line Seiberg index
What is the "Oreo cookie sign"?	When damaged dye enters Subchondral bone under talar dome 2/2 ankle injury
What is the normal lateral talocalcaneal angle?	CIA + talar declination angle = 45 degrees
What is eburnation?	subchondral sclerosis at cartilage erosion
What is TE (echo time) and TR (repetition time) in MRI? What are their trends in T1 vs T2?	Both inc (LONG) in T2 Both dec (SHORT) in T1 TR: REPITITION time, for T1 TE: ECHO time, for T2
What are the planes of imaging used in ultrasound?	Longitudinal and transverse
What is described as a "serpiginous" bone lesion?	Bone infarction, **osteonecrosis**
What are some comments you would make when reading an XR with an HAV deformity?	**1st MTPJ pathology** MAA structural deformity? TC CCA TN articulation Atavistic cuneiform 1st IMA TSP

	HAA PASA/DASA HIA **1st MT length compared** Seiberg MPE?
What are some comments you would make when reading a lateral view XR with a flatfoot deformity?	There appears to be a mild/moderate/severe structural flatfoot deformity as noted by a decrease in CIA 1) TC INC 2) Talar dec INC Cyma line ANT BREAK 3) Kirby sign 5) 1st MT declination (combined) DECREASED OPTIONAL: 6) LATERAL talo 1st MT angle if NC fault noted!! Seiberg index Fault
What are some comments you would make when reading an AP view XR with a flatfoot deformity?	1) TC 2) CAA 3) Talar uncovering **4) Forefoot adductus angle**
What is normal FF adductus angle? What is the effect with pronation?	<10 degrees DECREASES with pronation
What are some comments to make on an XR other than radiographic angles?	Soft tissue density Soft tissue contour follows underlying structures Break in cortices Bone density Joint congruity Joint space Osteophyte/ankylosis
What is Simon's angle?	Talo 1st MT
What is the range of normal CIA	18-30 or 24.5
What are the ranges of mild, moderate, and severe planus?	**Mild** 18-24 **Moderate** 10-18 **Severe** <10
What are some "structural" radiographic angles	IMA, CIA, MAA
What are some "positional" radiographic angles	HAA, TSP, Meary's, Seiberg's index, 1st MT dec, 5th MT dec
What is Toygar's angle with an Achilles rupture?	<150
What is the forefoot adductus angle? Normal? What is	FF to RF, normal 0-10, slightly less than MAA

the effect in pronation/supination?	pron-decrease, supination-increase
What is the lesser tarsus abductus angle? AKA? What is the effect in pronation/supination?	AKA lesser tarsus angle, midfoot to RF, pronation-inc, supination-decrease
From birth to 4 years, what is the order bones ossify?	0 year-cuboid (birth) 1 year-lateral cuneiform, 2 year-medial cuneiform, 3 year-intermediate cuneiform, 4 year-navicular
In regards to radiography, what is kVp?	peak kilovoltage the energy of electrons determining the maximum voltage across XR tube controls the **contrast**
In regards to radiography, what is mAs?	miliampere second, primary controlling factor of radiographic **density** and photon #
What is normal metatarsus adductus angle?	<15
how to draw talocrural angle, normal?	Tibial plafond and distal tips of malleoli normal is 8-15 or >83
What is normal Fowler Phillip angle?	<75
What is normal Hibb's angle?	1st MT calcaneus angle, >150
What is normal Kite's angle?	20-40, or 18
How does one decrease radiation when taking XR?	increasing KVP, decrease mA
What is X-ray fidelity? How does one achieve the best fidelity?	fidelity is the true size of original object, keep object as close to film as possible
How does one take a take medial and lateral oblique XR?	beam at 45 degrees medial oblique-medial foot planted on surface lateral oblique-lateral foot planted on surface
What is the Broden view? How does one obtain that view?	Views anterior—>posterior portions of posterior facet of STJ Knee flexed, foot internally rotated 45 degrees, X-ray beam with 10, 20, 30, 40 cephalic tilt
What is SID in X-ray terminology?	source to image receptor distance, distance between radiation source and radiation detector. smaller SID = increase density
What is OID in X-ray terminology?	object to image distance
What is the ossicle at medial malleolus?	os sub tibiale

What is normal talar declination?	21
When does navicular ossify? What else ossifies at this time?	4 yo, also lesser MT heads, base of phalanges
What is the purpose of developing of film? Uses what chemical?	change silver from **exposed** silver to **metallic** silver. use hydroquinone
What does kVp control? What is its effect on: Contrast? Quality? Exposure? **Penetration**? **Optical density?**	contrast (quality) increased kVp INC penetration, blacker **LOWERS** contrast, **LOWERS exposure** to patient, lowers XR quality
What does mA control? What is its effect on brightness and exposure to patient?	mA controls density, blackening of XR (quantity) increased mA INC XR brightness, inc EXPOSURE to patient
Where to aim X-ray beam in a medial oblique XR	lateral cuneiform
Where to aim X-ray beam in a lateral oblique XR	navicular
What is the Comma sign?	CN bar

Biomechanics

QUESTION	ANSWER
List some materials used to make orthotics	Polypropylene, graphite, carbon fiber
List some materials used to make cushioning in orthotics	Plastizote, neoprene, EVA
Semirigid vs rigid orthoses are good for what type of activities?	Semi-rigid: multidirectional (partially deform under WB) Rigid orthoses: unidirectional activities
Describe the difference between open cell vs closed cell orthotic cushioning	Open cell-collapses (poron) Closed cell-absorbs shock (plastizote)
what is a UCBL (University of California Biomechanics Laboratory) type of orthoses?	Deep heel cup + med/lat flange to restrict motion For severe flatfoot
Describe hip and knee range of motion during STANCE and SWING	Hip- stance (extend) swing (flex) Knee-stance (flex) swing (extends)
In limb length discrepancies, describe the effect on lumbar spine, shoulder drop, head tilt	Lumbar spine-convex towards SHORT side Shoulder-dropped on LONG side Head-tilted towards LONG side

Describe the range of motion of the 5th ray	Same as STJ (DMD to PLP), TRIPLANAR
In shoe anatomy, what is the "shank"?	Stiff inflexible material from heel center to ball of shoe to give support to longitudinal arch
In shoe anatomy, what is the "vamp"?	Forepart of shoe over toes and MT
In shoe anatomy, what is the "cookie"?	Stiff insert under arch
In shoe anatomy, what is the "last"?	Wooden or plastic model around which shoe constructed
Femoral retroversion/anteversion occurs in which plane? Which direction results in in-toeing?	Femoral head and neck in FRONTAL plane Retroversion: internally rotated→in-toeing
How does forefoot valgus compensate?	Longitudinal axis MTJ supination, STJ supination, oblique axis MTJ supination, STJ supination "LA SOS"
How to is tibial varum measured?	Inward angulation of distal 1/3 tib shaft toward NCSP
Foam cast for what type of deformity? Makes what type of orthotics?	Rigid deformities, accommodative orthotics
Describe the difference between open kinetic chain (OKC) movement vs closed kinetic chain (CKC) movement	OKC: movement around a joint that is NWB, calcaneus moves around talus which acts as extension of leg CKC: movement around a joint that is WB, both calcaneus and talus move
Describe pronation in OKC vs CKC	OKC: eversion, abduction, DF CKC: eversion, adduction, PF, tibia int rotates
Describe supination in OKC vs CKC	OKC: inversion, adduction, PF CKC: inversion, abduction, DF, tib ext rotates
If the direction of STJ moves towards the vertical, transverse, frontal positions, there is an increased deformity in which planes?	Vertical→transverse Transverse→frontal Frontal→saggital
In the gait cycle, how much time is spent in contact, midstance, and propulsion?	30%, 40%, 30% contact-heel strike to FF loading midstance-FF loading to toe off propulsion-toe off to heel strike
Describe the two parts of the swing phase of gait	First half-OKC pronation: help foot clear ground Second half-OKC supination: prepare for heel strike
What is the MC cause of FF varus? What is the MC cause FF valgus?	FF varus: lack of VALGUS talar torsion during development FF valgus: Weak TA, strong PL, PF 1st ray, weak

	post mm
List some types of AFO	Posterior leaf splint Solid-stops PF, limits DF, dropfoot pt with unstable knee Short leg with fixed hinge (Richie brace)-dropfoot pt with flatfoot, prevent internal rotation Dorsiflexion assist-moderate dropfoot Plantarflexory stop-prevent PF but normal DF
What happens to the degree of deformity if the STJ moves more vertically vs transversely?	vertically-increased transverse plane deformity transversely-frontal plane deformity
Tibial varum and tibial valgum's effect on RCSP	Varum –inversion Valgum—eversion
Describe the biomechanical function of the peroneus longus	Locks the medial column for added stability, leading to eversion of foot
How do you calculate RCSP?	RF varus MINUS STJ pronation
What is the "reverse windlass mechanism"?	Flat arch = plantarflexed hallux. Windlass unable engage, **unable to overcome GRF on first ray**, and foot unable to resupinate
How do you calculate resting calcaneal stance position (RCSP)?	**Varus NCSP:** calculate total amount of eversion by adding eversion and STJ neutral value **Valgus NCSP:** if >/=3, will drive calcaneus to "end of its ROM", or total eversion – amount tibial varum if </=2, NCSP does not change
How does forefoot varus compensate? What type of orthotic needed?	>/=3, STJ maximally pronates to end ROM </= 2, STJ pronates to RECTUS STJ will PRONATE so therefore, need a RF VARUS post
What causes an "abductory twist?"	1) FF varus, 2) compensation for a flexible FF valgus, 3) partial compensation RF varus
What are the stages of an abductory twist?	1. valgus FF, GRF pushes it into FF varus 2. STJ **pronates in late midstance→propulsion** to get FF and medial column back to the ground
What is the orientation of the STJ axis vs 1st ray axis?	STJ: distal medial dorsal (DMD)→proximal lateral plantar (PLP) 1st ray: distal lateral dorsal (DLD)→ proximal medial plantar (PMP)
What plane is the 1st ray **axis** in? What plane is 1st ray **motion** in?	**Axis**: TRANSVERSE **Motion**: FRONTAL and SAGGITAL, 45 degrees from

How many deg from these two planes?	these 2 planes
What is the MC cause of FF varus? What is the MC cause of FF valgus?	**FF varus:** lack of VALGUS talar torsion during development **FF valgus: Weak TA, strong PL**, PF 1st ray, weak post mm
How does equinus cause a hallux abductovalgus deformity?	0) Christensen et al first ray series in JFAS stated that equinus **INVERTS** the 1st MT and reduces the pull of PL 1) Increased FF loading causes instability of PL 2) Foot overpronates to compensate for lack of ankle DF 3) hypermobile first ray
List some types of AFO	**Posterior leaf splint** **Solid**-stops PF, limits DF, dropfoot pt with unstable knee **Short leg with fixed hinge (Richie brace)**-dropfoot pt with flatfoot, prevent internal rotation **Dorsiflexion assist**-moderate dropfoot **PF stop**-prevent PF but normal DF
List 5 types of functional compenstion for equinus	1. Abductory twist 2. Pronation of STJ 3. Knee flexion 4. Genu recurvatum 5. DECREASED stride length
How does the foot compensate for RF varus?	If enough pronatory movement to perpendicular = able to compensate Not enough motion = abductory twist
In limb length discrepanices, what is the effect in the following: lumbar spine, shoulder drop, head tilt?	**Lumbar spine**-convex towards SHORT side **Shoulder**-dropped on LONG side **Head**-tilted towards LONG side
What are some etiologies of equinus?	NM (CP), Osseus (arthritis, cavus), DM, congenital (normal), biomech (tight gastroc soleus)
Scissors gait is seen with which neuromuscular disorder?	Cerebral palsy
What is the most common cause of forefoot varus?	Lack of valgus rotation of talar head and neck during development, disrupting MTJ axis
What is the difference between a plantarflexed 1st ray vs forefoot valgus?	Determined by ROM of 1st ray: **Normal ROM** 1st ray = FF valgus **Restricted DF** 1st ray = PF 1st ray
What is the minimum ankle ROM necessary for gait?	10 degrees ankle DF, 20 degrees ankle PF

What is the minimum STJ ROM necessary for gait?	12 degrees total ROM
What is the difference between functional vs accommodative inserts	accomodative-plastizote, gel inserts funcitonal-rigid, put foot in STJ neutral
What is the McPoil tissue stress theory?	orthotics should reduce tissue stress rather than "deformities" of the lower extremity
What is the difference between forefoot supinatus vs forefoot varus?	**supinatus**-reducible, due to STJ pronation, affects MTJ, TRIplanar **forefoot varus**-nonreducible, causes STJ pronation, affects forefoot, frontal plane
What is Total Angle of Vega? When is it pathological?	Fowler Philip angle + CIA, pathological when >90
What is the normal STJ ROM?	42 from transverse plane 16 from sagittal plane
What is the windlass mechanism?	DF of the the MTPJ tightens the plantar fascia and raises medial longitudinal arch
Describe the progression of knee position from birth	varum (birth) —> straight —> valgum —> straight —> valgum —> straight
How many degrees minimum of STJ ROM needed for ambulation?	12 deg
How many degrees of extension is present in genu recurvatum?	>10 deg, can be due to limited ankle DF
What is the femoral angle of inclination? Birth vs adults?	axis of neck with shaft, Birth: 160 Adults: 127
What is the result of coxa vara/valga on the femoral angle of inclination?	vara: INC femoral angle of inclination valga: DEC femoral angle of inclination
What is the angle of declination of the femur?	AKA antetorsion, angle of femoral torsion, coronal axis of neck with distal condyles, Normal in adults: 6 degrees
What is the angle of anteversion of the femur?	angle of **femoral neck with pelvis**
What is tibial torsion? What is the normal value in adults?	lateral twist of tibia, angle of **malleolar position and knee axis adults: 20**
How is tibial varum/valgum measured?	Distal 1/3 leg perpendicular to ground and tibia
How many mm of LLD to cause functional/structural problems?	5mm
At what age does scoliosis appear in LLD?	13-14 yo
Which anterior leg muscle does not fire during swing?	peroneus tertius

What is a Thomas heel orthotic modification?	anteromedial extension to support longitudinal arch and limit pronation
What is a Dancer's pad orthotic modification?	offload 1st MT head, tx **sesamoiditis** or fractured sesamoid
What is a SACH heel orthotic modification?	round heel in rocker bottom fashion
What is a Denver bar orthotic modification?	under MT to support transverse arch
What is a cobra pad orthotic modification?	offload heel, fit into dress shoes
Describe scissor gait, seen with which neuromuscular disease?	aka **spastic gait**, internal rotation, adduction, dragging distal lateral foot seen with **CP**
Describe steppage gait, seen with which neuromuscular disease?	swing phase drop foot seen with **CMT**, guillain barre, CVA
Describe ataxic gait, seen with which neuromuscular disease?	instability during single limb stance. LOOK DRUNK seen with **MS**
Describe fenestrating gait, seen with which neuromuscular disease?	AKA shuffling gait seen with **Parkinson's**
Describe trendelenburg gait, seen with which neuromuscular disease?	contralateral tilt of pelvis seen with LLD, dislocated hip or **weak gluteus medius**
Describe dyskinetic gait, seen with which neuromuscular disease?	WRITHING gait, HYPERkinetic, high degree of variability **Huntington's chorea**
Describe vaulting gait, seen with which neuromuscular disease?	**Steppage of the side with prosthesis** Myotonic dystrophy
Describe hemiplegic gait	Circumduction of hemiparetic side

Medications and Anesthesia

QUESTION	ANSWER
What is the antidote for acetaminophen toxicity?	n-acetylcysteine
Which Inhaled anesthetic sensitizes myocardium?	halothane
What part of spinal cord does one inject spinal anesthesia?	subarachnoid space
What are the side effects of an ester vs amide	ester-more prone to allergy, amide-toxicity

Which spinal structure does one pierce when performing a spinal block?	Arachnoid
What is the MOA of bisphosphonates	Induces apoptosis of osteoclast
How does one calculate creatine clearance in men vs women?	Cockcroft gault equation: **Men:** (140 − age) x weight / 72 x creatinine **Women:** multiply by 0.85
What is voltaren? What 2 factors make it unique from other drugs in its class?	Diclofenac AKA arthrotec when combined with misoprostol **Unique**-GI protection, inhibits COX AND LOX
Which NSAID is sulfa drug?	Celecoxib
What is the dosing of LMWH?	1mg/kg SC Q12
What is the MOA of Sulfonylureas? What are some examples?	MOA: **INCREASE** insulin secretion from pancreatic beta islet cell *"urinate out a tide of insulin"* Glyburide, glipizide
What is the MOA of biguanides? What are some examples?	MOA: inhibit glyconeogenesis in liver, **INCREASE** insulin sensitivity *"met the big foreman who is very sensitive to insulin"* Metformin (Glucophage)
When is antibiotic peak measured? How how is it adjusted?	30 min AFTER 3rd dose, adjust by inc dose
When is antibiotic trough measured? How is it adjusted?	30 min BEFORE 4th dose, adjust by timing
What is the maximum does of acetaminophen?	4000mg / day
What is the antidote for opioid toxicity?	narcan AKA naloxone
List some examples for oral narcotics	hydrocodone, oxycodone, morphine, percocet
Heparin vs coumadin—intrinsic vs extrinsic pathway?	heparin-intrinsic coumadin-extrinsic
What is the MOA of loop diuretics? Name some	MOA: inhibits NaCl at ascending limb, STRONGER i.e. furosemide
What is the MOA of potassium sparing diuretics? Name some	MOA: inhibits K+/Na+ channel at collecting tubule i.e. spironolactone
What is the MOA of thiazide diuretics?	inhibit NaCl at ascending loop and distal convoluted tubule
What are some side effects of antipsychotics?	parkinsonian syndrome, tardive dyskinesia

What is hyaluronidase? What is its MOA?	fibrolytic that **breaks down connective scar tissue** and allows for increased dispersion of IV medication throughout the tissues.
What is APAP or acetyl-para-aminophenol?	Tylenol AKA acetaminophen or paracetamol
What are some side effects of tramadol?	N/V, lower seizure threshold
What is nabumetone?	AKA **RELAFEN**, only non-acidic, alkaline NSAID, selective COX2
What is the antidote for CO poisoning?	100% O2
Name a topical NSAID	Diclofenac
What are 2 names for topical treatments for MRSA?	Bactroban (mupriocin)
What drugs increase PT/INR?	Antibiotics due to vitamin K alteration in gut flora
Name an IV NSAID. What is its maximum length of administration?	Ketorolac (toradol) 5 days max due to kidney damage
Which type of diuretic is used for patients with gout?	K+ sparing, spironolactone
Name some side effects of Lamisil	Abdominal pain (RUQ), jaundice
What is the dosing for Lamisil?	250mg QD x 90 days
Name the difference between tramadol vs toradol	toradol (ketorolac) is IV NSAID tramadol is for opioid allergy
Name some oral narcotics	hydrocodone, oxycodone, morphine, percocet
What is bleomycin used for?	Removal of warts
What are some side effects of NSAIDs other than GI bleed?	Caution in asthmatics-COX inhibition increases leukotriene production, a bronchoconstrictor
What are some narcotic options for patients with opioid allergy?	STUD: stadol, toradol, ultram, darvocet
Why does lidocaine act faster than marcaine?	closer to body's pH, but also results in faster metabolism
Which antihyperglycemic drug is contraindicated with IV contrast?	Metformin (renal failure)
Name 3 anti-laxatives	imodium (loperamide) opioids
Name 3 anti-diarrheals	colace (docusate) dulcolax (bisacodyl) milk of magnesia(magnesium hydroxide)

What is the maximum dose of Zofran?	4-8mg Q8
What type of local anesthetic is used after popliteal block?	0.25% marcaine
What is a common side effect from opioids (not constipation)? What is its treatment?	itching give hydroxyzine
What are some side effects of steroids (injection vs oral)?	**injection**: skin necrosis, steroid flare, skin/fat atrophy, hypersensitivity, hypo pigmentation **oral**: adrenal suppression, impaired wound healing, imparied bone healing, Cushing's syndrome, hyperglycemia
What is the dosing of naproxen?	250mg BID
What is the dosing of motrin/ibuprofen?	400mg Q6
What is another name for these following anticoagulants: lovenox, arixtra, trental, plavix, pradaxa?	Lovenox = enoxaparin Arixtra = fondaparinux Trental = pentoxifylline Plavix = clopidogrel pradaxa = dabigatran (A fib)
What is the mechanism of action of terbinafine vs griseofulvin?	**terbinafine**: inhibits squalene epoxidase, prevent metabolism of squalene to lanosterol/ergosterol preventing cell wall synth **griseofulvin**: binds to microtubule to inhibit mitosis
What is the only NONREVERSIBLE NSAID?	aspirin
How are oral steroids dosed?	need to wean off to prevent addison like symptoms due to negative feedback
Which local anesthetic can be used when a patient is allergic to an amine and ester?	benadryl (diphenhydramine)
Name the antidote for anticholinesterase (physostigmine, neostigmine)	atropine (ACLS)
Name the antidote for benzodiazepine	Flumazenil
Name the antidote for digoxin	digoxin immune antibody
Name the antidote for methanol	ethanol
Name the antidote for iron	deferoxamine
Name the antidote for lead	succimer (DMSA)
Name the antidote for methotrexate	leucovorin calcium (folinic acid)

Name the antidote for tricyclic antidepressants	physostigmine
Name 2 uses for mucomyst	AKA n-acetylcysteine, for acetaminophen OD and for renal protective agent after radioactive dye
Which diuretic is not good for patients with gout?	loop diuretics (furosemide) due to inc uric acid
Which drug for rheumatoid arthritis is also used in treatment of malaria?	plaquenil, aka hydroxychloroquine
What is the most common drug combination to cause malignant hyperthermia?	halothane + succinylcholine
Name the 4 classes of NSAIDs	salicyclic acid, proprionic acid, acetic acid, oxicam
Describe the difference between ester and amides in terms of length, metabolism, and side effects	ester-detox in blood, shorter, anaphylaxis amide-detox in liver, longer
Mechanism of action of local anasthetics	decreases permeability of Na+ ions to block nerve conduction
What is the mechanism of action of coumadin? How is it reversed?	extrinsic pathway 2, 7, 9, 10. Reverse with vitamin K and fresh frozen plasma
What is the dosing for vicodin?	5/300 or 5/500
What are 2 contraindications for an anesthetic with epinephrine?	Allergy and thyrotoxicosis
Name some side effects of ketamine	Increased blood pressure, increased salivation, increased CSF
Where is spinal anesthesia administered?	AKA subarachnoid block, administered n subarachnoid space, through dura and arachnoid below L2 to avoid spinal cord
What are the most common drugs used in spinal anesthesia?	Marcaine with epinephrine
What are some side effects found with spinal anesthesia?	headache 2/2 loss of CSF thru meningeal needle hole, dec buoyancy of brain. Difficult to control. HYPOTENSION 2/2 sympathetic depression, URINE RETENTION
What is neuroleptic anesthesia?	Light general anesthesia or "cognitive dissocation"
Which 3 anesthesia drugs have no analgesic effect?	Etomidate, midazolam, barbituates
What are some side effects of succinylcholine? What is used to treat toxicity?	Side effect: myalgia Antidote: neostigmine
What is the mechanism of action of local anesthetics?	Inhibit nerve conduction by inhibiting Na+ channels to INCREASE THRESHOLD for depolarization

What is a side effect of all inhaled anesthetics?	Increases bronchial secretion. Halothane prevents secretions (serves as bronchodilator)
Which drug decreases respiratory tract secretions?	Anticholinergics (atropine, scopolamine diphenhydramine)
Which fluoroquinolone should be used with caution in asthmatics?	Ciprofloxacin
Name some examples of mild, moderate, and potent grades of steroids	**mild**-hydrocortisone **mod**-triamcinolone **potent**-betamethasone, clobetasol
What is atropine used for?	dilate pupil, decrease secretions
What is a side effect of quinines? What is it used for?	Used to treat arrhythmias, antimalarial Side effect: Cinchonism (ringing in ears, deafness)
Salicyclic acid is toxic at what concentration?	>6% destroys tissue
What is podophyllum used for?	Wart treatment, antimitotic agent
What is procainamide used for?	Antiarrhythmics
What is the warfarin loading dose?	10mg PO x 2 days
What is the dosing of colchicine and mechanism of action?	0.5-1g inhibits neutrophil from phagocytosis urate crystal

Procedures & Surgical Technique

QUESTION	ANSWER
Which steroids are injected into the joint vs soft tissue?	Kenalog (acetate) in soft tissue, a precipitate Dexamethasone (phosphate) used in joint
Name the only nerve not blocked by popliteal block	Saphenous (comes off femoral)
At what point does anterior tibial artery become dorsalis pedis artery?	After crossing inferior extensor retinaculum
What is a Loeffler-Ballard incision?	begins at 1st interspace along medial arch to medial malleolus to expose all 5 central plantar spaces
What is an Ollier incision?	Incision over lateral STJ used in excision of CN bar, triple arthrodesis
Name 2 styles of tendon lengthening	Z-plasty, accordion type lengthening

Hardware

QUESTION	ANSWER
Name 3 reasons to countersink a screw	Prevent stress fx, soft tissue irritation, even compression
Name the least reactive suture to tissue	prolene
What is a Herbert screw?	headless screw proximal and distal threads separated by smooth shaft. Leading threads have greater pitch. Provides some compression, can be inserted through cartilage
What is the "Rule of 2's" in regards to screw fixation?	2 threads, 2 finger tightness, 2x length to width, 2 pts of fixation
List some methods for tendon fixation	Bone anchor **Trephine plug**-using cortical bone **Button anchor** Tunnel with sling **Tendon with bony insertion** Mason allen stitch-1) horizontal 2) vertical over **Screw and washer** **Chinese finger trap**-draw tendon through a drill hole
List some absorbable skin sutures. Which suture is the longest acting?	Polyglactin 910 (Vicryl) Polydioxanone (PDS) Monocril (Poliglecaprone) **Polyglyconate** (Maxone) longest acting "MAX" Polyglycoic acid (PGA)
What type of metal should be used in talar fracture fixation?	Titanium so MRI can be used to r/o AVN
Describe the "stress shielding concept"	All internal fixation absorbs physiological stress so bone will resorb (Wolff's law)
What is an interference screw?	Fully threaded headless screw w/o compression to prevent axial displacement
Detritic synovitis is a foreign body reaction to what material?	Foreign body reaction to shards of **silicone**
Name the 4 components of stainless steel. Which component prevents breakdown? Which component gives hardness?	Iron, **chrome** (prevents breakdown), nickel (allergy), **carbon** (gives hardness)

What are 2 benefits of titanium hardware?	Very inert, good for MRI
What is the tension stress effect?	For lengthening with external fixator, **distraction at proper rate will lead to tissue growth**
What is Hook's law?	The force needed to extend/compress a certain distance is proportional to that distance
What screw sizes would you find in a **mini** frag set and what are their underdrill values?	Underdrill values in parentheses: 1.5 (1.1), 2.0 (1.5), 2.7 (2.0)
What screw sizes would you find in a **small** frag set and what are their underdrill values?	Underdrill values in parentheses: 3.5 (2.5), 4.0 (2.5)
What screw sizes would you find in a **large** frag set and what are their underdrill values?	Underdrill values in parentheses: 4.5 (3.2), 6.5 (3.2)
What does "lag by design" mean?	Partial threaded screw
What is a bridging plate?	Neutralization plate without interfrag screw
What is the weakest part of screw?	Runout (where threads start)
List the steps for proper AO screw insertion	underdrill (predrill) distal cortex over drill proximal cortex countersink measure tap insert
How is the overdrill is for a threaded screw determined?	TRICK question, no overdrill is needed for threaded screws
How are 2 screws oriented to fixate a fracture?	1 perpendicular to fx line 1 perpendicular to shaft of bone
How is 1 screw oriented to fixate a fracture?	Halfway between shaft and fx line
What is NITINOL?	"Nickel Titanium Naval Ordinance Lab" A malleable metal made of nickel and titanium, solidifies at body temp
How many screws and cortices are needed to fixate the syndesmosis?	2 screws across 3 cortices OR 1 screw across 4 cortices
List some examples of suture anchors	Arthrex ® speed bridge, harpoon anchor, Mitek ®, corkscrew,
What is the function of a hook plate?	Secures small medial malleolar fragments
Describe how to fixate the medial malleolus	4.0 cancellous, or malleolar screw, perpendicular to fracture line and parallel

What size are syndesmotic screws?	3.5 or 4.5
At what level relative to the ankle joint are syndesmotic screws placed? What is the risk?	2 and 4 cm proximal to ankle joint, the 4cm likely to hit perforating peroneal A
List some examples of absorbable and nonabsorbable suture	**absorbable**-polyglactin, polyglecaprone, POLYDIOXANONE (PDS) **nonabsorbable**-polyester, polypropylene, nylon, silk
What is Vicryl made of? When does it lose its strength?	Vicrly AKA polyglactin 910 65% tensile strength at 14 days hydrolyzed in 3-4 months
What is the width of saw blade called?	Kerf
How does one manually tap a screw?	2 forward rotations, 1 backward rotation (to remove thread bits)
List the K-wire sizes and their relative diameters in milimeters	.28, .35, .45 (1.1 diameter), .54 (1.4 diameter), .62 (1.6 diameter)
What k-wire can you use to under drill a 1.5mm screw?	4-5 kwire (0.045 inches or 1.1 mm)
What is the purpose of lag technique? How does bone heal	generates compression which leads to immobilization. Bone heals by **immobilization**, not compression
List some techniques to prevent thermal necrosis of the drill bit	sharp tip, fast advancement, slow drill speed, firm force
What is monocril?	Monocril AKA poliglecaprone dissolves in 20-30% tensile strength @ 2 wks hydrolyzed in 3-4 months
What is a dynamic compression plate?	Oval, sloped, deeper holes enabling eccentric drilling and axial compression
What is a neutralization plate?	Redistribution of force through plate + interfrag compression.
What is a buttress plate?	uses tension force on convex side of injury
What is limited contact plate?	grooves on underside of plate to limit periosteal contact
What is a malleolar screw?	partially threaded self cutting cortical screw
What is fiberwire?	polyethylene multifilament core + braided polyester jacket
What is ethibond?	braided polyester (nonabsorbable) used for tendon repair

What is the purpose of tapping a screw?	tap cuts threads in bone to allow torque applied during screw insertion to generate compressive force instead of being dissipated by friction.
How do you calculate the size to tap a screw	Same as overdrill size
Do cancellous screws need to be tapped?	no
What is the design of self-tapping screws?	fluted tips, which should be advanced beyond distal cortex
What is lysophilization?	freeze drying (allograft)
What is screw pitch?	distance between threads
How does tension band fixation work?	reverses tension on convex side into compression
What type of screws for triple arthrodesis?	6.5 or 7.0 cannulated
What is the strongest suture with longest absorption rate?	stainless steel
What are the 4 priniciples of AO technique	Anatomic Reduction, Early ROM, atraumatic dissection, stable fixation
What does AO stand for? What does ASIF stand for?	Arbeitsgemeinschaft fur Osteosynthesefragen, Association for the study of internal fixation
What is the difference between lag by design and lag by technique?	Lag by design is a partially threaded screw designed to only purchase the far cortex. Lag technqiue you overdrill the near cortex for a fully threaded screw.

Pre, Intra, & Post-operative

QUESTION	ANSWER
What is normal INR? What is the cutoff value for surgery?	normal: 1 surgical cutoff: <1.4
What value of HCT is the cutoff for surgery?	< 24%
Toxic dose of lidocaine in a 70kg patient? With and without epinephrine?	300 plain or 500 with epi 7mg/kg with epi 5mg/kg plain
Toxic dose of marcaine in a 70kg patient? With and without epinephrine?	175 plain or 225 with epi 3mg/kg with epi, 2mg/kg plain
Is lidocaine more or less toxic with epinephrine?	LESS toxic because vasoconstriction prevents it from spreading to soft tissue and heart

Lidocaine with epi vs lidocaine plain, which one do you need more to to achieve equivalent anesthetic effect?	MORE needed with regular lidocaine. Lido with epinephrine shortens onset and prolongs effect
What is normal HCT	40
List the causes of post op fever in order of acuity of presentation	Wind water walking wound wonder
What is normal pre-albumin?	30
What is the minimum hemoglobin required for surgery?	>10
What does SCIP stand for?	Surgical Care Improvement Program
According to SCIP, when are antibiotics necessary?	TKA, THA
Within how many hours are perioperative antibiotics administered?	within 1 hr of tourniquet time
When are 2 grams of ancef necessary instead of 1g?	If pt >175lbs
How far to stand from sterile field (when not scrubbed in)?	1 foot
What are the maximum ankle and thigh tourniquet pressures?	Ankle: no greater 125-150mmHg, 250mmHg max. Thigh max 500mmHg Deflate after 2 hrs for at least 15-20 mins
List 4 antiemetics	zofran (odansetron) 4-8mg Q8 reglan (metaclopramide) phenergan (promethazine) zyprexa (olanzapine)
List 3 anti diarrheals	colace (docusate) dulcolax (bisacodyl) milk of magnesia(magnesium hydroxide)
What are the guidelines for NPO status?	no solid food/milk 6-8 hrs before clear liquid okay 2-4 hrs before
What is the treatment for malignant hypothermia?	dantrolene
What is the normal hemoglobin in males vs females? What is the minimum required for surgery?	Male-14-18, Female-12-16, 10 for surg
What are the INR values for elective vs emergent surgery?	Elective-1.3, emergent-2.3
What are some physical exam tests to rule out DVT?	Pratt's test-squeeze calf Homan-DF foot

What are the laboratory findings to indicate malnutrition	Albumin: Norm >3.5 g/dl, mild malnutrition 3-3.5g/dl, moderate malnutrition 2.5-3 g/dl, severe malnutrition: <2.5 g/dl
What are some options to treat white toe, from least to most invasive?	drop the foot, loosen dressing, warm compress, massage toe, rotate K-wire, remove sutures, nitropaste vasodilation (could lead to hypotension), lidocaine plain injection, remove pin.
What is the minimum distance between two skin incisions to avoid necrosis?	1cm
What are risk factors for DVT formation?	**S-STASIS** (immobilization) **H-HYPERCOAGULABLE STATE** (obese, birth control) E-**ENDOTHELIAL INJURY** (smoking, Factor 5 leiden defect)
What is the name of the PE/DVT clinical assessment score?	Wells score/criteria
What are some causes for hemoglobin/hematocrit to drop?	Surgery, antibiotics, blood draws, hypercoagulable states, anemia
What causes malignant hyperthermia? What is the treatment?	reaction to anesthesia—halothane and succinycholine. treatment: stop anesthesia, get creatine kinase, 100% O2, cool down, dantrolene sodium
What are normal values for PT/PTT?	PT: 10-13, PTT: 24-34
What are some causes for postoperative pain after foot and ankle surgery?	sutures tight, dressings tight, hematoma, ischemia, compartment syndrome, edema
What are some causes of a nonhealing surgical wound?	mal-aligned with resting skin-tension lines, infection, steroids, desiccation (dry), alcoholic malnutrition
What are some reasons to prescribe post op antibiotics?	history of previous infection, medical comorbidities, history of wound healing difficulty
Wwhat percent of DVT—> PE	25%
Name contraindications for tourniquet use	infection, PVD, compartment syndrome, Raynaud, DVT, recent bypass
when to d/c anticoagulants before surgery, when to resume?	d/c 3-6 days before surgery, resume 24 hrs post op

ASA surgical risk classification	1-healthy 2-mild dz (DM, HTN) 3-severe activity limiting dz (angina, COPD) 4-life threatening dz 5-pt not expected to survive 24 hrs 6-organ harvest
When is it appropriate to stop coumadin prior to surgery?	3 days, switch to heparin drip, stop 2-4 hrs pre surgery
How long is surgery supposed to be postponed after MI?	6 months
List some indications to give antibiotics for endocarditis prophylaxis	valvular heart disease, rheumatic murmur, prosthetic valve
Which of the 5 W's of post-op fever occurs the earliest?	WIND-ateletasis and aspiration pneumonia occur 24-48 hrs where others are 72+ hrs
How long does a popliteal block provide anesthesia?	14 hours
What are the benefits of using an ankle tourniquet over a thigh tourniquet?	less pain, less DVT
What is the purpose of subchondral drilling?	increases surface area for fusion, allows for vascular bridging and bone formation

Plastic Surgery

QUESTION	ANSWER
Describe a partial thickness skin graft and its source What is done about the donor site?	PART of dermis taken from gluteal region can leave donor site OPEN
Describe a full thickness skin graft and its source What is done about the donor site?	ENTIRE dermis Taken from groin/flexor surface in a **3:1 ratio** CLOSE donor site primarily
What is a stent dressing?	hold graft in place, pressure, absorb fluids
List some causes for graft failure	seroma, hematoma (MC), infection, shearing, poor prep of recipient site
How is the incision oriented to de-rotate an adductovarus deformity of the 5th toe?	distal medial —> proximal lateral. Perform a concomitant arthroplasty
What is a Cincinatti incision?	transverse incision across Achilles

The lateral extensile incision outlines which artery?	peroneal artery

Bioinformatics

QUESTION	ANSWER
Positive predictive value (PPV) vs negative predictive value (NPV)	PPV = true positive / all positives NPV = true negatives / all negatives
Ordinal	Order matters (visual analog scale)
Nominal	No order (name only, i.e. blood type)
Interval	Inherent order with defined interval (temperature)
Calibration vs discrimination	Calibration-risk representing group Discrimination-risk representing individual
Absolute vs relative risk	Absolute-group Relative-individual (25x)
Principal of equipoise	ethical when there's no clear evidence one is better than other
Hawthorne effect	patients perform differently when being experimented on
Efficacy	treatment under IDEAL circumstance
Effectiveness	treatment under REALITY
type 1 error	false **positive**
type 2 error	false **negative**
Parametric test	follows BELL CURVE
length time bias	Identify diseases with inherent good prognosis i.e. screening for breast CA
Standard error of mean	Estimate of **standard deviation** by taking a smaller sample size

Medicine

QUESTION	ANSWER
List 3 types of anemia	Micro <90, iron def Normo 90-100, chronic Macro >100 B12, folate
Describe the Parkland formula	Calculate the amount of resuscitative fluid for the first 24 hrs to keep burn patient hemodynamically stable 4mg/kg (lactated ringer) x %burned first half in 8 hrs, remainder over 16 hrs (lactated ringer w/o dextrose for first 24hrs, THEN protein and dextrose)
What is rhabdomyolysis?	Damaged skeletal mm tissue are released into bloodstream and cause kidney failure **Exertional**: heat illness, seizure, **Non-exertional:** alcoholism, weight lifting, steroid use, protein
What are the function of the posterior, lateral, anterior columns of the spinal cord?	Lateral-pain/temp Posterior-vibration/proprioception Anterior-light touch
What causes typhus?	Rickettsia
Name the tick causing Rocky mountain spotted fever	Wood tick
In a patient with HTN, which medication can be continued during surgery?	Beta blocker
In a patient with RA, which medication can be continued during surgery?	Prednisone
Name the drug of choice for syphilis	PEN G or doxycycline
What are some of the early laboratory signs of diabetes? (other than glucose or HgbA1c)	Microalbuminuria >100
How is DM2 diagnosed?	Fasting glucose >120 x2 or nonfasting >200 or HbA1c 6.5-7
At what blood sugar do you start dumping sugar in urine?	BS > 200, 250 is when affects wound healing
What is the triad for Felty's Syndrome?	RA, neutropenia, splenomegaly
List another name for osteitis deformans	Paget's disease

What is mycosis fungoides?	Cutaneous T cell lymphoma

Anatomy

QUESTION	ANSWER
Describe the ligaments of the Lisfranc complex	Dorsal, plantar interosseus (strongest) DORSAL weakest. NO Intermetatarsal ligament
What are the 3 arteries that supply the base of the 5th metatarsal?	Periosteal arteries, nutrient arteries, metatarsal arteries, epiphyseal metaphyseal
Describe the rotation of the Achilles tendon as it inserts onto the posterior calcaneus	12-15cm from insertion, rotates 90 deg COUNTERCLOCKWISE ROTATION med fibers→ posterior posterior fibers → lateral
What is Baxter's nerve?	Nerve between FDB and quadratus plantae Also the nerve that goes to abductor digiti minimi
Where do lateral and medial bands of the plantar fascia insert?	Lateral-base of 5th Medial-no insertion
List the borders of the popliteal fossa	Semimembranosus-proximal medial Biceps femoris-proximal lateral Distal-gastroc heads + plantaris (laterally)
What is the blood supply for the sural muscle?	Sural arteries
What is the origin/insertion of the plantaris muscle?	Origin: lateral femoral condyle Insertion: at medial Achilles
What is the difference between a sesamoid vs accessory bone	Sesamoid-within tendon or joint capsule Accessory bone-does not have to be in tendon/joint capsule
What is the source of the popliteal artery?	Superficial femoral
Describe the origin and insertion of the long plantar ligament	Calc to MT base 2-5
Describe the origin and insertion of the short plantar ligament	Calc to cuboid
Name the origin of the muscles in the anterior compartment of the leg (TA, EDL, EHL)	TA-tib EDL-tibfib inteross EHL-inteross fibula
Describe the dorsal arteries of the toes	dorsal MT arteries —> dorsal digital proper arteries

Describe the plantar arteries of the toes	plantar MT arteries —> plantar digital proper arteries all come from lateral plantar except 1st plantar digital proper
What is the normal diameter of the Achilles tendon?	LESS THAN 6mm
What is the function of spring ligament?	support talar head, medial arch stabilization
Describe the difference between Morton's vs Joplin's neuroma	**Morton**-3rd IM space, **Joplin**-medial 1st MPJ
Where does peroneus tertius insert?	base of 5th MT
Function of superficial and deep deltoid	superficial-prevent eversion deep-prevent axial rotation
What is another name for Lemont's nerve?	Intermediate dorsal cutaneous
Name the tendon medial to EHL	extensor hallucis capsularis (88%)
What is the ligament of Lazaro known as?	fibulotalocalcaneal ligament
What is the depth of the 1st TMT jt	3.2cm
Which muscles insert on base of proximal phalanx of hallux?	aDDuctor hallucis, aBDuctor hallucis, FHB, EHB, plantar fascia
Describe the blood supply to head/neck, body, posterior of talus	head/neck-DP, ant tib body-A of tarsal canal (PT) A of sinus tarsi (peroneal A) posterior-calcaneal branches of PT, peroneal A
Name the nerve root for the medial and lateral plantar nerves	L4 L5
Where does the EDL insert?	extensor expansion
What is the function of extensor hallucis capsularis?	Stabilize 1st MTPJ, take away slack upon DF
List the attachments to base of 5th MT	Lateral band plantar fascia, PB, **Flexor digiti minimi brevis**-originates on base of 5th MT, inserts on base of 5th toe
Name the strongest deltoid ligagment	Tibiocalcaneal ligament
Where does the peroneal N cross fibula? Where does the sural N cross Achilles?	Peroneal N: 7cm prox to fibular tip Sural: 9.83cm from insertion
Name the strongest syndesmosis ligament	PITFL (42%) of syndesmotic component
Name the deepest part of deltoid ligament	deep anterior talotibial ligament
What is the crural cruciate ligament also known as?	INFERIOR extensor retinaculum

What is the transverse crural ligament also known as?	SUPERIOR extensor retinaculum
What nerves join to make the sural nerve?	1) tibial nerve—>medial sural cutaneous 2) peroneal nerve—> sural communicating branch
Which joint in foot is saddle shaped?	CCJ
At which digit do the medial and plantar cutaneous nerves split their innervation?	Plantarly-4th digit Dorsally-3rd digit

List the components of popliteal artery trifurcation	Popliteal
	    1) anterior tib (becomes PTA)
	    2) circumflex fib A
	    3) peroneal A

List the 9 compartments of the foot	4 interossei, medial, lateral, central superifical, central central, central deep
List the muscles found in superficial/deep central, medial lateral compartments	**Superficial**-FDB **Deep**-adductor hallucis **Medial**-abductor hallucis **Lateral**-abductor digiti minimi
Where do flexor digit minimi brevis and abductor digiti minimi insert?	Base of 5th DIGIT ORIGIN of FDMbrevis on base of 5th MT
Describe the foot dermatomes dorsally and plantarly	**Dorsal**: L4 L5 medial, S1/S2 lateral (sural) **plantar**: same for forefoot, S1/S2 heels
Name the components of the floor and roof of porta pedis	floor-abductor hallucis, roof-quadratus planate
What is the Lacinate ligament also known as?	flexor retinaculum
Describe the blood flow from the aorta to big toe	Aorta aortic arch descending aorta abdominal aorta common iliac, external iliac femoral superficial femoral, popliteal tibio-peroneal trunk anterior tibial DP **1st dorsal MT, proper dorsal digital A**
Which nerve most likely injured from surgical repair of Achilles tendon?	Sural N
Describe the course of superficial peroneal nerve	in lateral compartment between PB/PL mm bellies, pierces fascia cruris to innervate dorsal foot
Which toe is innervated by two different nerves DORSALLY? PLANTARLY?	**DORSAL**: 3rd toe (medial AND intermediate dorsal cutaneous) **PLANTAR**: 4th toe (med/lat plantar)

What layer is medial plantar nerve located in? Lateral plantar nerve?	medial-1st, lateral-beween 1st and 2nd
How many bones, how many joints in foot?	26 bones, 33 joints
List the layers of foot	1-"hang loose sign" abductor hallucis, FDB, abductor digiti minimi 2-"wave bye bye!" QP, lumbricals 3-"hold up 3 fingers" adductor hallucis, flexor digiti minimi, FHB 4-interossei
What is the function of the long and short plantar ligament?	Supports the lateral column
What does the tibial N divide into at the foot?	medial/lateral plantar, medial calcaneal branches
List the borders of tarsal tunnel	medial-flexor retinaculum lateral-talus, calcaneus anterior-medial malleolus
Describe the innervation of muscles in the plantar foot[1]	medial plantar: "LAFF": lumbrical 1, abductor hallucis, FDB, FHB everything else is lateral plantar
List the nerves blocked in ankle block	"PSST": peroneals (deep and superficial) saphenous, sural, tibial
List the lumbar root of femoral nerve, sciatic, tibial	femoral: L2-L4 sciatic: L4/5 S1-3 tibial: same as sciatic
List the borders of femoral triangle	Inguinal ligament Adductor longus Sartorius
Is the deep transverse MT ligament found superficial or deep to the nerve?	superficial
What structures make up the Lacinate ligament?	fascia crucis and deep transverse fascia
What is camper's chiasm?	split FDB which allow FLD to pass through
How many lumbricals are there, and where do they insert?	4 insert on medial prox phalanx. originate on medial FDL tendons
How many interossei are there and where do they insert?	**plantar**-unipennate, 3 on medial side 5, 4, 3 **dorsal**-bipennate, 4 insert on lateral side and both sides of 2nd

List the surgical layers of dissection	skin, superficial fascia (neurovascular structure), deep fascia (muscle, deep neurovascular), periosteum, bone
What are sharpey's fibers?	attach periosteum to bone
List the branches of the sural nerve	medial sural cutaneous of tibial N sural communicating (from lat sural cutaneous) of common peroneal N
What is saddle bone deformity?	metatarsal cuneiform exostosis
What is the cervical ligament of the foot also known as?	anterior talocalcaneal ligament
List the nerve root for saphenous, superficial peroneal, deep peroneal, sural nerve	saphenous: L3/L4 superficial peroneal: L4/L5 S1 deep peroneal: L5 S1/S2 sural: S1/S2
At what level does superficial peroneal cross fibula?	7cm proximal to fibular tip
List the attachments of the Lisfranc ligament	Strong interosseous lig connecting 1st cuneiform bone and the medial base of the 2nd met bone.
Name the sciatic nerve root	L4-S3 Sciatic foramen under piriformis mm
Where is the medial dorsal cutaneous N located on the dorsal foot?	Medial to EHL

Anesthesia

QUESTION	ANSWER
What percent of surgical cases are ASA (American Society of Anesthesiologists) risk category 1 or 2?	40-60%
1. What are some side effects of nitrous oxide? 2. What are some indications for use of nitrous oxide?	1. **Side effects:** BM DEPRESSION: pernicous anemia (BM suppression) from chronic exposure in office staff, least potent so low resp/cardiac SE . Give 100% O2 s/p surg to prevent hypoxia 2. **USE:** hx of malignant hyperthermia, rapid induction (low BGC)
At what ages should an EKG, CXR, and pregnancy test be obtained prior to surgery?	EKG: >40 yo Pregnancy test <50 yo CXR: >60 yo

What are some anesthesia risks for sickle cell patients?	hypoxia, low cardiac output, unstable BP
What is the "minimum alveolar concentration"?	Amount inhaled anesthetic at one atm that prevents movement and response to noxious stimulus in 50% of pts. LOW IS BETTER
What is the blood gas co-efficient?	Solubility of agent which determines speed of induction, emergence, dosing LOW IS BETTER, less amt needed
What is the use of an Infiltrative/field block?	Good for small area
1. What is Monitored anesthesia care (MAC) 2. What combination of drugs are used?	1. local anesthesia + conscious sedation, not necessarily safer, quicker recovery, no LOC 2. Remifentanil, midazolam (low resp depression, low N/V). Can also use propofol, midazolam, fenatnyl
What is the order of nerve fibers that are affected by local anesthetics?	Sympathetics>pain>temp>touch>proprioception >motor
What are 3 uses of a common peroneal N block?	1) ankle stress XR 2) dx peroneal spastic flatfoot 3) unable for distal blocks 2/2 trauma/infection
What are 2 contraindications for anesthetic with epinephrine?	Sensitivity and thyrotoxicosis
Which peripheral vessels are NOT innervated by sympathetic nerves?	Capillaries
Of all the anti-hypertensive medications (ACEi, B blocker, diuretics) which ones are held prior to surgery?	Hold diuretics only
When are antacids used in anesthesia?	Mg citrate, sodium citrate give 15-30 min prior to induction for emergency operations
What are some clinical warning signs of malignant hyperthermia	Claw clenching, muscle spasm, muscle wasting
What type of anesthesia can be given if patient has severe respiratory disease?	Spinal epidural or etomidate/thiopental sodium
What is the optimal positioning for obese patients?	Increase O2 demand decrease lung volume Lateral or supine position
What are some symptoms of sickle cell crisis? What is the treatment?	Fatigue, malaise, joint pain Treat with hydroxyurea
What body parts are at risk for injury in supine position?	Brachial nerve plexus –ULNAR nerve
What body parts are at risk for injury in prone position?	Eye socket and dorsum of foot

What is involved in mask induction?	Max gas flow using O2, NO and halothane (least resp tract irritation, less cough, less laryngospasm)
Which inhaled agent has the quickest emergence?	Isoflurane
What are some risks during emergence?	Vomiting, airway obstruction, laryngospasm
What are some anesthesia risks in diabetics?	Silent MI and autonomic dysfunction leading to hypotension and bradycardia
1. What region of the spine is epidural anesthesia administered? 2. What position is the patient put in? **3.** What are some side effects?	Continuous catheter, LARGER dose, LONGER onset 1. Epidural space short of dural mater at the cervical, thoracic or lumbar spine 2. Lateral prone position 3. SE: lower risk of headache unless puncture dura and enter subarachnoid
What is considered the "epidural space"?	Foramen magnum to coccyx
1. What layer of the region of the spine is spinal anesthesia administered? **2.** What drugs are used? **3.** What are some side effects?	AKA subarachnoid block, one time injection 1. In subarachnoid space, thru dura and arachnoid, below L2 to avoid spinal cord 2. MC: Marcaine with epinephrine, inc motor blockade and tolerance to tourniquet 3. **Side effects**: headache 2/2 loss of CSF thru meningeal needle hole, dec buoyancy of brain. Difficult to control. HYPOTENSION 2/2 sympathetic depression, URINE RETENTION
What are some indications for bier block?	General anesthesia risk, hx spinal arthritis
What is the preferred agent used in bier block?	Lidocaine w/o epi
What is the nerve root for the sciatic nerve?	L4-S3, passes through sciatic foramen under piriformis mm
What is the nerve root for the tibial nerve?	L4-S3
What is the nerve root for the common peroneal nerve?	L4-S2
Where is the injection made to block the superficial dorsal cutaneous N? What about to block the sural nerve?	**Superficial dorsal cutaneous N**-1cm above med mall at the ant ankle **sural N**-inferior to lateral mall
Where does the deep peroneal pass relative to other tendons as it crosses the ankle joint?	Between EDL and EHL (same as anterocentral port for arthroscopy)
Where is the saphenous N located relative to the	LATERAL to saphenous V

saphenous vein?	
How do locals cause vasodilation?	Block SYMPATHETIC nervous system
What is the "Lemont test"	Plantarflex and invert ankle to visualize intermed dorsal cut N
What is the MOA of benzodiazepines?	Facilitate GABA action by INC freq of Cl channel opening
What are the steps in performing a Bier block?	1. 1 tourniquet below knee, one below common peroneal N 2. Cannulate vein 3. Elevate limb to exsanguinate 4. Inflate proximal to 275-300 5. Administer lidocaine 3mg/kg 6. INFLATE distal when patient complains of pain, then RELEASE proximal
What is the mechanism of action of local anesthetics?	Inhibit nerve conduction by inhibiting Na+ channels to INCREASE THRESHOLD for depolarization
Which anesthetic's side effect involves retrograde amnesia? Which anesthetic's side effect involves dissociative anesthesia?	Retrograde amnesia: midazolam Dissociative anesthesia: ketamine
Which benzodiazepine has fastest onset?	Midazolam
Which inhaled drug increases the risk of arrhythmias?	Halothane-sensitized by catecholamines, the only nonvolatile agent (gas at room temp)

Grab Bag

QUESTION	ANSWER
Name two types of stents used in vascular surgery	drug eluting, bare metal
What are the differential diagnoses for leg pain?	DVT, rhabdomyolysis, compartment syndrome, necrotizing fasciitis
List the normal values for found in a Chem7 panel	sodium 135-150, potassium 3.2-5.2, chloride 95-110, CO2 20-30, BUN 5-25, creat 0.5-1.5
List the normal values found in a CBC	WBC 4-12, hb: 14-18 males, 12-16females, HCT: 40-55 males, 35-50 females, platelet 150-450K
Pre, intra, post renal azotemia	Pre: dehydration Intra: abx tox, glomeruli nephritis, post infect Post: obstruction

What is the MOA of allopurinol?	xanthine oxidase inhibitor
What is xanthine oxidase?	enzyme to breakdown purines into uric acid
What is the MOA of probenecid?	prevents reabosorption of uric acid @ proximal tubule
What lab values are used to calculate the LRINEC score?	glucose, WBC, creatinine, CRP, sodium, hemoglobin,
Describe the clinical triad for tetanus	trismus (lockjaw), risus sardonicus (face), aphagia
Describe the best location for plate placement in ORIF	tension side (plantar for MT shaft), but not possible due to mm
What is primaxin?	imipenem cilistatin
What is known as aviator's astralagus?	talar neck fracture due to forced DF
What is timentin?	ticarcillin clavulanate, anti pseudomonal
List some factors that can cause false negative value of CRP	normalizes with NSAID, ASA, steroid, oral contraceptive
Describe the 2 types of leukocytes	leukocyte (WBC) includes 1. **granulocyte**-neutrophil, eosinophil, basophil 2. **agranulocyte**-monocyte, lymphocte (viral infection or leukemia)
What is normal range of glucose?	80-120
List some gas forming bacteria	clostridium perfringens, bacterioides fragilis, peptostreptococcus
How is ESR measured?	the Westergren method, the distance erythrocytes fall in 1 hr in column of anti coagulated blood under influence of gravity. Dependent on amount of fibrinogen
Where along the 5th metatarsal is a Jones fracture typically located?	1.5cm proximal to 5th MT tuberosity
Why do you get equinovarus deformity with TMA?	lose long flexors and extensors which are the stabilizers of the foot (also lose PB)
Describe the Fallat classification for 5th MT Which is the most common?	1-enlarged head 2-lateral bowing 3-increased IMA 4-combined stage 4 inc IMA is most common
Typical clinical presentation for Freiberg's disease	young female athlete with MT pain

Name the most common osteochondrosis	Legg Calve Perthes disease, femoral head
Describe the classification for accessory navicular. Which one is the most common?	1-os tibiale externum 2-synchondrosis A-parallel, B-plantar 3-gorilloid navicular types 2 and 3 make 70%
At what point does open fracture change from contaminated to infected	untreated for 6-8 hrs
In joint-depression calcaneal fractures, does the Bohler/Gissane's angle increase or decrease?	Gissane-increase Bohler-decrease
What part of brain regulates temperature?	hypothalamus
List the stages of skin graft healing	1) plasmatic (fibrin anchor) 2) inosculation (re-vascularization) 3) reorganization re-innervation
Describe the pathophysiology that causes diabetic retinopathy and neprhopathy	accumulation of sorbitol from the polyol pathway. sorbitol cannot cross cell membrane so it draws water in, producing osmotic stress
Describe the MOA for erythromycin	50s
Describe the MOA for gentamycin	30s
Describe the MOA for vancomycin	bind to d-ala d-ala
What is the best imaging technique to differentiate between osteomyelitis and nonunion?	indium 111 WBC scan
Describe the mechanism of action for bactrim	inhibits bacterial folinic acid synthesis
Describe the microbe present from a dog bite	capnopcytophaga canismorsus
Describe how to convert HbA1c to average blood glucose	HgbA1C 7 = 140 glucose, add 20 for 1 pt HgbA1c
Name the temperature range that meets SIRS criteria in degrees Fahrenheit	min 96.8, max 100.4
Describe the difference between infant vs child vs adult osteomyelitis	**infant**-connection between metaphysis and epiphysis **child**-no connection **adult**-no physis
What is HOCM?	Hypertrophic cardiomyopathy, the leading case of sudden cardiac death in children. enlarged myocardium, alignment of muscle cells disrupted (myocardial disarray)

List the 4 generations of penicillin	1-penG, penV 2-nafcillin, oxacillin (PCNase resistant) 3-amoxicillin, ampcillin (aminoPCN) 4-pipercillin, ticarcillin (ext spectrum)
Describe the difference between a band cell vs PMN	band: immature WBC PMN: mature WBC
What is a "left shift"?	increase in band
For DM1 (IDDM) preoperatively, what type of insulin should be given?	1/3-1/2 of daily dose of intermediate insulin (NPH)
Name the most common microbe for vertebral osteomyelitis	Staph aureus
Increased cortical thickening is due to what hormone?	Growth hormone (acromegaly)
Ultrasound is not a good imaging choice in which instances?	Vascular disease, epiphysis (growth plate), infection, implants, pacemaker
List some contraindications for spinal anesthesia	Bleeding disorder, shock/hypovolemia, septicemia (risk meningtitis), neurologic disease (MS) or anything increasing ICP, cardiac disease, spinal deformity (back pain), intestinal perforation
Side effect of spinal anesthesia is headache due to puncture of what anatomical structure?	Puncture of dura, and enter subarachnoid space
What is the skin lesion diameter to diagnose melanoma?	**>6mm** (pencil eraser)
1) What is the next step in the presence of a 4mm raised PPD skin test? 2) If chest XR positive for TB, what is the next step?	1) CXR 2) RIPE treatment, isolation
What bug causes spinal infection post spinal anesthetic?	Neisseria meningitis
Which endocrine disease increases K+, dec Na+?	Addison's
What disease causes honeycomb bone lesion in skull?	thalassemia
Patient with recent MI with stent, presents with dyspnea, rales, LE edema, suspect what disease?	Right sided heart failure
Most common metatarsal to fracture?	5th MT
List all of the 12 cranial nerves	olfactory, optic, occulomotor, trochlear, trigeminal, abducens, facial, vestibulocochlear, glossopharyngeal, vagus, spinal accessory, hypoglossal

List the types of shock	hypovolemic, septic, cardiogenic, anaphylactic shock, neurogenic shock, obstructive shock
Describe the difference between hyponichium and eponychium	hypo-distal nail plate epo-proximal nail plate
Name the eponyms for 1st and 2nd interspace neuromas	Heuter-1st, Hauser-2nd
What is the clinical presentation of sickle cell anemia? How do the wounds appear? Is it autosomal dominant or recessive? Which microbe are these patients susceptible to? What causes aplastic crises and what is the treatment?	**CP**: long bone pain, arthralgia with fever, dactylitis, back, abdominal, limb pain, HEMATURIA, ASEPTIC NECROSIS OF HIPS **Wounds**: punched out lesions **Genetics**: autosomal recessive Bug: salmonella **Aplastic crises/aplastic anemia**: (PARVOVIRUS) infection —> stop produce RBC **Treatment**: FLUIDS, analgesics, hydroxyurea
What is the "female athlete triad"?	eating disorder, amenorrhea, osteoporosis
What is somatization disorder?	dramatic emotional complaints, vague, any part of body, dissatisfied with physician care
List the neuromuscular diseases to cause cavus foot	spinal bifida, CMT, Friedreichs, Polio, myelomeningocele, CP, syphilis
Name 2 oral drugs to treat psuedomonas	Ciprofloxacin and levofloxacin
Name the skin scraping test to diagnose nail fungus	KOH
In antibiotics, what is the role of cilistatin?	renal dihydropeptidase inhibitor to increase half life
D-test shows sensitivity to what antibiotic?	clindamycin
What is the workup for a patient who presents with stable angina with normal EKG?	stress test, echo, angiography
Where are langerhans cells located and what is their function?	Throughout epidermis, function as macrophage (immune system)
What are the function of melanocytes?	Basal cells, produce melanin to absorbe UV light
Describe erythema nodosum and erythema multiforme	**Nodosum**: Inflammatory skin lesion on SHINS, SARCOIDOSIS, ulcerative colitis **Multiforme**: deposition of IgM, MUCOSAL MEMBRANE, 2/2 drug reaction (Steven Johnsons) or infection
How is Seiberg's index of the 1st MT measured?	Difference between the distance between MT necks and MT base 1.5cm distal to MCJ
What value of D dimer may suggest DVT?	D dimer >500

What is post phlebitic syndrome?	s/p DVT, LE edema 2/2 to incompetent valve
List 4 examples of primary HYPERthyroidism	Graves, toxic mutlinodular goiter, thyrotoxicosis, thyroid storm
List 2 examples of primary HYPOthyroidism	Hashimotos: nonpainful, rubbery, symmetrical Subacute thyroiditis: PAINFUL, enlarged, asymmetrical Radioactive thyroid ablation, litihum, iodide
Describe the order of ossification of bones in the foot pre-birth	MT→phalanges→calc→ talus→ (cuboid)
Describe the 4 types of nevus	1) **Blue**: Failure of **melanocytes** from nerves to arrive at dermo-epidermal jcn. Melanocytes remain at lower dermis. 2) **Junctional**: demo epidermal jcn, most likely→melanoma 3) **Compound**: dermo-epidermal jcn AND dermis 4) **Intradermal**: dermis ONLY
Which skin lesion is described as a "strawberry mark"?	Capillary hemangioma
Describe renal failure (pre, intra, post)	**Pre**: dehydration, infection, blood loss, hypotension, HTN **Intra**: glomerulonephritis, drugs, ATN (most problematic) **Post**: enlarged prostate, stone
Describe molluscum contagiosum	Pox virus, pearly umbilicated papular epithelial lesions, inclusion bodies
Why is TBI a more accurate better test than ABI?	TBI b/c digital vv do not have tunica media, will not be falsely elevated 2/2 calcification
List some non absorbable skin sutures	Prolene (polypropylene)-least reactive, good for infection Nylon Polyester (Teflon) Polybutester Silk, fiberwire (not for skin)
Describe clinical findings of sarcoidosis	**Non caseating granuloma in lung**, SOB, non productive cough, **erythema nodosum**
Name the term used to describe pain from non-painful stimuli	Allodynia
What is another name for the peroneal stop procedure	PL to PB tenodesis
Syncope tx	Lay flat, loosen neckwear

List some symptoms for diabetic ketoacidosis (DKA)	**DKA**: DM1 Orthostatic hypotension, tachycardia, Kussmaul breathing, fruity breath, DEHYDRATED Tx: fluids, K+, insulin BS 350-900 **Hyperosmolar coma**: DM2, NO ACIDOSIS
What are some symptoms of malignant hyperthermia? What is the treatment?	Fasciculations, **jaw clenching**, rigidity, hyperthermia due to EXCESSIVE RELEASE of Ca2+ from sarcoplasmic reticulum. Dantrolene **prevents** Ca2+ release
In the administration of local anesthetics, how is toxicity differentiated from anaphylaxis?	**Anaphylaxis**: reaction with para-aminobenzoic acid (PABA) **Toxicity**: CNS stimulation FIRST (tinnitus, metallic taste, numb mouth), then CV: myocardial depression, bradycardia
What is an anaphylactoid reaction?	Anaphylaxis after first exposure, does **NOT** require sensitization Dose-related toxic mechanism
Where is a glomus tumor located?	Subungual nail bed
What is the treatment for hypoglycemic syncope?	25cc 50% dextrose IV, or give orange juice if conscious
Fibrosarcoma risks metastasis to which organ?	Lung
What is the limiting factor in lengthening a short metatarsal?	Vascular length
What are the MC causes of Charcot foot?	**Syringomyelia**-cyst in spine & **diabetes** **Tabes dorsalis (syphyllis)**, spina bifida, CMT
What are meniscoid bodies?	Synovial villi hypertrophy in ankle arthroscopy
What is the side effect of digitalis? Which lab value needs to be monitored?	Arrhythmias, monitor K+
What is pterygium?	overgrowth of LUNULA (or conjunctiva in eye)
What can cause oily nail?	Psoriasis, papulosquamous disorder
What is the microbial coverage of clindamycin?	Gram positive, gram negative, anaerobe
Describe the difference between immediate type hypersensitivity vs delayed	**Immediate**: IgE dependent release from sensitized basophil and mast cells after contact to allergen **Delayed**: T-cell mediated
Pheochromocytoma is a tumor of which organ? What are some associated symptoms?	Tumor of adrenal medulla secreting epinephrine and NE Symtpoms: HTN, flushing, headache

What is a therapeutic use of anabolic steroids? What are some side effects?	Use: Relieve bone pain in osteoporosis SE: alopecia, HTN, sterility
List some side effects of barbiturates	Dec in BP and compensatory inc HR, porphyria
Why isn't it appropriate to give high doses of insulin for treatment of DKA?	Insulin will drive K+ into cell → hypokalemia
What is the range of fluid capacity in a bladder?	400-600cc
In a growth plate, which zone is the weakest region?	Zone of maturation (hypertrophic)
List 5 bone tumors that can have a soap bubble appearance	Giant cell, ABC, hemangioma, non ossifying fibroma (fibrocortical defect), chondromyxoid fibroma
CPK can be released from comes from which organs?	Skeletal mm, heart, brain
What is the posterior column portion of the spinal cord responsible for?	Sensory-vibration, proprioception, position
What is the extrapyramidal portion of the spinal cord responsible for?	Reflexes, coordination, balance *"it takes coordination to build a pyramid"*
What is the corticospinal portion of the spinal cord responsible for?	contralateral side
What is the lateral spinothalamic portion of the spinal cord responsible for?	Pain and temp
What is the advantage of the prone suspension technique for casting orthotics?	FF to RF relationship can be visualized from behind, manipulate STJ
What are some uses for ultrasound therapy in treating musculoskeletal injuries?	Reduce tightness and spasms, decrease inflammation, assist healing
How is infant mortality rate calculated?	#deaths/#live births (expressed out of 1000)
What are low risk methods for DVT prophylaxis?	Stockings or SCD (sequential compression device)
What is the purpose of lidocaine in ACLS?	Suppress PVC's **(premature ventricular contractions)**
What is the function of the State department of health?	Public health policies and standards, collect, analyze, and disseminate health information
What are some symptoms of sepsis in an elderly patient?	Urinary incontinence, dehydration, respiratory alkalosis, increased respiratory rate
What are some risk factors for Kaposi's sarcoma?	African, immunosuppressed, AIDS
List Breslow's depth	1. <.75mm 2. .75-1.5mm 3. 1.5-3mm

	4. >3mm
In screw anatomy, what is known as the "land"?	Underside of head to contact cortex
In screw anatomy, what is known as the "shank"?	Unthreaded portion of screw
In screw anatomy, what is known as the "pitch"?	Distance between threads
What is a risk factor for basal cell carcinoma (BCC)?	Sun exposure
List some suture patterns for repair of Achilles tendon rupture	Krackow-interlocking Bunnell-figure of 8 or weave Kessler-box
List some methods for Achilles augmentation/lengthening	FHL, plantaris, gastroc aponeurosis, fascia lata, V→Y lengthening, Graft jacket (allograft dermal derivative), Pegasus (equine pericardium)
List some risk factors for tendon rupture	Age (decreased elasticity), Xanthoma (hyperlipidemia), steroid injection
Describe the ASA surgical wound classification	1-clean uninfected 2-clean contaminated (resp/GI/GU tract) 3-contaminated (fresh wound, break in sterile technique 4-dirty (existing infection)
What are some contraindications for bier block?	Allergy to local, previous thrombophlebitis, vein stripping, infection
What are some clinical differences between right and left sided heart failure?	**R side**: LE edema, hepatomegaly, JVD **L side**: tachypnea, rales/crackles, pulmonary edema,
In the treatment for brachymetarsia, where is the osteotomy placed for callus distraction?	Proximal **metaphysis**
What is the maximum dose of acetaminophen vs ibuprofen	Acetaminophen-4000mg Ibuprofen-3200mg
List the pros and cons of propofol	Pro: fast induction, euphoria, Con: greater CV/resp depression
What is the roentgen equivalent in man (REM)?	Radiation in workers 1mrem/h = 2000 mrem/yr
What are contraindications to MRI?	Certain implants that are magnetic
List the 4 types of types of onychomycosis, and infectious agent	1. Distal subungual (DLSO)-MC, T. rubrum 2. White superficial (WSO)-**T. mentagrpphytes** 3. Proximal subungual (PSO)-**immunocompromised**, T. rubrum

	4. Candida-water
Describe the difference between basal vs prandial insulin	Basal-low rate of continuous insulin, adjusted based on activity (**Lantus** or **levemir**, LONG or INTERMEDIATE acting) Prandial- prior to meal (**human insulin, aspart, lispro**, FAST acting)
List some options for topical hemostatic	Gelfoam, **topical thrombin**, bone wax
How is pulmonary embolism diagnosed?	Clinical symptoms, D dimer, CT angio, VQ scan, **EKG (r/o cardiac ET),** echo
Describe the two types of COPD	Obstructive lung disease 1) **emphysema-**pink puffer 2) **chronic bronchitis-**blue bloater, ANKLE SWELLING
In a gram stain, what color denotes gram positive vs gram negative organisms?	Gram positive - PURPLE Gram negative - PINK
List some gram + cocci (aerobic) What is microbe is known as group D strep (GDS)?	Staph aureus, staph epi, strep (**B hemolytic**: GAS s pyogenes, GBS s agalactiae), strep viridans (**alpha hemolytic**), ENTEROCOCCUS (**gamma hemolytic**) (VRE) Group D strep (GDS) - strep bovis
List some gram + cocci (anaerobic)	Peptostreptococcus, peptococcus
List some gram + rod (aerobic)	Bacillus anthracis, **corynebacter** (diptheriae, **minutissum**), listeria
List some gram + rod (anaerobic)	Clostridium spp (perfringens, dificile, botulinum)
List some gram – rod (aerobic)	Pseudomonas, (HEN PECKSS), vibrio vulnificus, enterobacter, eikenella, pasturella, Yersinia pestis
List some gram - rod (anaerobe)	B frag, fusobacter
List some gram - cocci (aerobe)	Neisseria
List some spirochetes	Treponema pallidum, borellia burgdorferi
Describe the difference between how a serous vs hemorrhagic fracture blister forms	**Serous-**fluid within epidermis **Hemorrhagic-**fluid between dermal epidermal junction
Describe 2 types of incisions for ORIF of calcaneal fracture	1) lateral extensile 2) minimally invasive via arthroscopy
At what spinal level is spinal anesthetic placed?	L4-L5
What is the difference between sensitivity vs specificity?	Sensitivity: how well will capture positive Specificity: how well will NOT capture negative

When can a mitral valve prolapse heard?	mid systolic, increases with valsalva maneuver
HLA B27 is positive in what conditions?	Reiters disease, ankylosing spondylitis, psoriatic arthritis, ulcerative colitis
Rheumatoid factor is positive in what conditions?	RA, SLE, Sjogren
List some extra-intestinal symptoms of ulcerative colitis	Iritis/uveitis, arthritis, erythema nodosum
Describe the difference between a static vs dynamic compression plate	**Static**-eccentric drilling **Dynamic**-place on tension side of bone. WB will increase compression force
What are the different ranges availble for compression stockings	16-18-DVT ppx 25-35-venous insufficiency 40-50-lymphedema
How does hyperbaric oxygen therapy (HBOT) work?	Chamber of 100% O2 at 2-2.4 atm for 90 min, TCOM (transcutaneous oxygen monitoring) to increases from **30-40 to >200** Angiogenesis and fibroblast production to help collagen synth and epithelial closure
How much compression is provded by a Profore® dressing?	40mmHg at ankle, 17mmHg at calf
What is the function of an alginate dressing?	Highly absorbent and for bleeding areas
Describe 2 types of classification systems for osteomyelitis	1. **Waldvogel and Lew**-chronicity 2. **Cierny Mader**-anatomic type (medullary, superficial, diffuse, etc), host (immune system), and systemic factors
What is the protocol if the capital fragment is dropped onto the floor during a bunionectomy?	5 minutes of betadine cleanse followed by saline rinse
What disease would you find a "Port wine stain"	Sturge weber
Describe what you would see on XRay vs MRI for an Achilles rupture	**X-Ray**-radiodense gap, soft tissue edema, obliteration of kager's triangle **MRI**-wavy tendon = retraction of tendon, hyperintense signal around tendon 2/2 hematoma
List some Indications for surgical treatment of Achilles rupture	Delayed tx >2-4wks, elderly, medical co-morbidities, ATHLETES
Describe the difference between hyaline vs fibrocartilage	Hyaline-type 2 cartilage Fibrocartilage-mixed type 1 and type 2 cartilage
What metallic component of stainless screw can cause an allergy?	Nickel
What is the Rumpel leede test?	Tourniquet test to assess for capillary fragility

What is the pathogenesis of osteogenesis imperfecta?	Malfunction in type 1 collagen production
What are some symptoms for common Iliac A obstruction?	Weak femoral pulse, sexual dysfunction, buttock claudication
List some symptoms of hyperthyroidism	Lid lag, warm moist skin, fine tremors
A lower motor neuron (LMN) lesion would result in what type of gait?	Steppage gait
What is the treatment for Gustillo Anderson stage 3?	1) OR I&D with ex fix and CULTURES 2) Return to OR once cultures are negative
How is a posterolateral approach directed in order to fix posterior malleolar fracture?	Between Achilles and peroneal tendon
Difference between mechanism of injury between Jones fracture vs 5th MT base avulsion fracture	**Jones**-5th MT base remains fixed with internal rotation of foot **Avulsion fracture**-lateral band of plantar fascia
List 4 different fixation options for ORIF of Jones fracture	1) **4.5 cancellous fully threaded** with lag technique 2) ex fix with mini rail 3) tension band wiring 4) dynamic compression plate
What are 2 indictions for ORIF of Jones fracture?	Delayed presentation, athlete
1. Describe the "homerun screw" used to fixate a LIsfranc fracture 2. What is the surgical goal in fixation of Lisfranc injuries? 3. When is conservative treatment okay in Lisfranc injuries?	1. Home run screw from medial cuneiform to base of 2nd MT 2. Surgical goal: reduction and stabilization of medial and central columns 3. Conservative okay if <2mm displacement
What is the normal prealbumin level?	20-40
What is the protocol for tetanus vaccine?	Toxid **every 10 yrs** Toxoid is the booster. If unknown, give 250cc immunoglobulin
What is the most common direction of displacement of the 2nd metatarsal in a Lisfranc injury?	DORSAL and LATERAL
Describe cerebral palsy	NONPROGRESSIVE BRAIN LESION altering motor control disorder in movement and posture
Describe erythromelagia	Neuropathic pain syndrome resulting in HYPEREMIC skin reaction. NOT a seronegative arthropathy
Which Salter fracture is through the physis?	Salter 1

Rheumatic fever attacks which heart valve?	Mitral valve
Describe risk factors and clinical apperance of basal cell carcinoma (BCC)	SUN Exposure, (umbilicated) central ulceration dry and crusted, BLEED on debridement
Describe the clotting factors involved in the intrinsic vs extrinsic pathways, vitamin K, and common pathway	**Intrinsic (PTT):** 8 9 11 12 **Extrinsic (PT):** 3 7 **Vit K:** 2 7 9 10 **Common:** 1 2 5 10 13
Does an accessory navicular CAUSE flatfoot?	No
What is the proper position to fuse the ankle?	Neutral and 5 degrees valgus
Describe peudoequinus	Limited ankle DF due to rigid PF nature of FF
Which component of the deltoid ligament is the strongest?	Tibiocalcaneal ligament
What can cause blue nail?	Minocycline or SILVER nitrate exposure
What is the direction of the osteotomy for the Weil procedure?	Distal dorsal to plantar prox
What constitutes a positive lachman stress test?	2mm or >50% dorsal displacement
What are some factors that cause impaired wound healing in diabetics?	Increased inflammatory phase, decreased vasculature, decreased collagen synthesis
What is the effect of diabetes on tendons and joint capsule?	Non enzymatic glycosylation leads to stiffness
What class of anti-HTN medications can cause hyperglycemia?	THIAZIDE
What is the surgical cutoff for BUN/creatinine	BUN 50 creat 3
What are the vital signs of shock? What is the treatment goal?	**INC HR/RR**, dec H/H, dec cap fill, **DEC urinary output**, Mental status change GOAL: restore organ perfusion
Who first described Charcot disease?	Musgrave 1703 JM Charcot (tabes dorsalis syphilis) in 1868
In the neurovascular theory of Charcot there are damages to which part of spinal cord?	DM damages trophic centers in anterior horn leading to increased blood flow and osteoclast activity
What are the 3 MC causes of Charcot disease?	Syringomyelia, DM, tabes dorsalis Other: myelomeningiocele, spina bifida, CMT, MS, CP, polio, TB, **trauma to brian/spinal cord**
In XR findings for Charcot disease, will you find atrophic or hypertrophic bone formation?	**BOTH** **Atrophic**-osteopenia, bone resorption

	Hypertrophic-deposition, fragmentation, debris
How often should XR be taken to follow up Charcot disease?	4-6 wks
List the microbes known as the human mouth pathogens	HACEK Haemophilus, actinobacillus, eikenella, **kingella kingae**
What are the factors that make up the mangled extremity severity score (MESS)?	Ischemia, age, shock, mechanism of injury Significant score if 7 or higher
List some examples of alpha vs beta hemolytic step	**Alpha**-viridans, pneumo **Beta hemolytic**-GAS/GBS
What is the minimum size of glass to be visible on XR?	>5mm
What are some indications for a foreign body be removed?	Infection, **contaminated** object, pain, close to NV elements, intra-articular
Who first described a Jones fracture?	Robert Jones while ballroom dancing
Describe the mechanism of injury for a Stewart type 2 5th MT fracture?	Shearing force with contracture of PB
What are the XR findings for a Torg stage 3 5th MT fracture?	Obliteration of IM canal
Describe the steps performed in ORIF of a Lisfranc fracture dislocation	1) Homerun screw, 2) 2nd MT→intermed cuneiform, 3) 3rd MT→lat cuneiform 4) 0.062 k wire thru 4th and 5th MT thru cuboid
What is another name for a Destot fracture?	Trimalleolar fracture
What is BUN?	Protein metabolic waste product produced by liver
Describe the mechanism of action of thiazolidinediones	Increased cellular response to insulin -ZONE
List some rapid, intermediate, short, and long insulin types	Rapid-lispro (Humalog) aspart (novalog) Intermediate-NPH, lente Short acting-regular Long-lantus glargine, levemir
What are some causes of fever up to 107, 105 degrees?	107-anesthetic hyperthermia 105-blood transfusion reaction
What is the difference between thread diameter vs core diameter?	**Thread**-overdrill **Core**-underdrill (shank) diameter w/o threads
What is Vicryl hydrolyzed into?	CO_2 and H_2O

What is Lister's corn?	5th digit DIPJ, PIPJ, lateral nail fold
What is the Koebner phenomenon indicative of?	Psoriasis, skin lesion along lines of trauma
What drugs give metallic taste?	Flagyl, lamasil, local anesthetic
What organ breaks down glucocorticoids?	Liver
What is the difference between Raynaud's phenomenon and Raynaud's syndrome	**Phenomenon**-cyanosis **Syndrome**-recurrence of phenomenon 2/2 to collagen or autoimmune disorder, cold, emotion
What is the MC symptom of lymphatic obstruction?	NON-pitting edema
List some bacteriocidal antibiotics	Those that destroy cell wall- beta lactam, Vancomycin, Cephalosporins, , Carbapenem, Fluoroquinolone, metronidazole, monobactam, daptomycin
List some bacteriostatic antibiotics	BACTRIM, CLINDAMYCIN, TETRACYCLINE, MACROLIDES, tigecycline
What are some causes for anion gap metabolic acidosis?	MUDPILES Methanol, uremia, DKA, polypropylene glycol, infection, lactate, ethanol, salicylates
What is Steida's process known as?	Posterolateral process of talus
What are some symptoms of adrenal crisis?	Severe abdominal/lower back pain Increased Ca2+, low BP, low glucose Due to **low cortisol 2/2 untreated Addison's**
What is the difference between hypertensive urgency, emergency, and crisis?	**urgency**-high BP >220/120, **emergency**- + symptoms **crisis**- + organ damage
What are 3 etiologies of nyastagmus?	1. CNS-vertigo (central-brain vs peripheral-vestibulocochlear) 2. Toxic/metabolic 3. Multiple sclerosis
What is the best lab test for RA?	Anti CCP most sensitive
What is the imaging of choice to diagnose pulmonary embolism?	CT angiography
What do increases and decreases in alkaline phosphatase indicate?	**decreased**: hypoTH, malnutrition **increased**: liver and bone disease, hyperPTH, normal children's growing bones
In diabetics, what is the "Dawn phenomenon"?	elevated blood sugar in AM due to waning insulin and GH surge
In diabetics, what is the "Soymogyi effect"?	**REBOUND HYPERglycemia** due to overnight

	hypoglycemia (unrelated to insulin)
Adrenal insufficiency, 2 causes, which MC?	**Primary**-MC, due to ADDISONS **Secondary**-due to abrupt cessation of steroid treatment
Describe giant cell arteritis: 1) Which vessels does it affect? 2) What is the clinical presentation? 3) What is the treatment?	1) Affects large and medium vv, esp EXT CAROTID A 2) Temporal headache, jaw pain, visual disturb 3) steroids (glucocorticoids)
What does a holosystolic heart murmur suggest?	Mitral and tricusp regurgitation
What does a decrescendo heart murmur suggest?	Pulmonic/aortic regurgitation
What does a crescendo decrescendo heart murmur suggest?	Pulmonic/aortic stenosis
Describe the treatment for subungual hematoma	<25% trephination >25% remove nail
Who can waive doctor patient priviledge	Patient only, Written consent required for doctor to invoke legal privilege on patient's behalf (disclose information)
4 elements of tort	Duty, breach, causation, damages
What is capitation?	Fixed periodic HMO payment calculated to cover the expected cost of providing services to pts over a period of time

21499913R00054

Printed in Great Britain
by Amazon